Psychoanalysis and Analytic Psychotherapy in Japan

Psychoanalysis and Analytic Psychotherapy in Japan

By

Takayuki Kinugasa

Translator: Ms. Masayo Hasuda

Cambridge
Scholars
Publishing

Psychoanalysis and Analytic Psychotherapy in Japan

By Takayuki Kinugasa

This book first published 2022

Cambridge Scholars Publishing

Lady Stephenson Library, Newcastle upon Tyne, NE6 2PA, UK

British Library Cataloguing in Publication Data
A catalogue record for this book is available from the British Library

ISBN (10): 1-5275-8141-1
ISBN (13): 978-1-5275-8141-8

TABLE OF CONTENTS

ON DISORDERS

CHAPTER 1

STUDIES ON NARCISSISM IN THE UNITED KINGDOM: ESPECIALLY ON KLEINIAN STUDIES

I would like to present my studies on narcissism in the United Kingdom.

In the United Kingdom, there are few patients who fall into the classification of patients with the American narcissistic personality, and there are many patients with a schizoid personality or borderline personality. The study of narcissism in the United Kingdom developed as a study of the narcissistic organization seen in these patients or psychotic patients. It was the Kleinians, especially H. Rosenfeld, who mainly studied it. I would like to summarize the representative papers by Rosenfeld and then present an actual clinical case of mine.

As for the studies by the British Independent Group in London, there is the study of D. W. Winnicott on the development of normal narcissism under the "holding" situation, and the study of "false self" as its pathology. There are also the studies of M. Balint, that is, criticism on Freud's primary narcissism and the study on basic fault. However, it was Rosenfeld and other Kleinian analysts who most systematically addressed the issue of narcissism. Therefore, this paper will focus on Rosenfeld's research and describe the development of studies on narcissism in the United Kingdom.

Rosenfeld addressed the issue of narcissism in his paper in 1964, "On the Psychopathology of Narcissism: A Clinical Approach". What he focused on was narcissistic transference in therapy and he discussed its dynamics. He examined patients with dispositions of narcissism in general but some of them were considered to be patients with a schizoid personality and some were patients diagnosed with schizophrenia. Probably, within that broad spectrum, patients with narcissistic personality who are studied in the United States were included. In his paper, Rosenfeld considers as follows:

Freud classified his patients, in his paper in 1914, into patients with transference neurosis and patients with narcissistic neurosis, and he included patients with dementia praecox in the latter, which is a group of patients who do not develop transference. They show resistance like a stone wall, do not show interest in the therapist, and are considered incurable.

However, therapists of such severe patients, especially patients with schizophrenia, ignore Freud's distinction between transference neurosis and narcissistic neurosis, and consider that narcissistic neurosis does cause transference and that the transference is primitive. They also state that transference of narcissistic neurosis is truly narcissistic and the analyst and patient's self fuse, or features such as primitive destructiveness and extreme idealization of analysis can be seen.

Rosenfeld points out that such pioneers do not distinguish primary narcissism and secondary narcissism, as Freud distinguished, in narcissistic transference. He also considers that their clinical descriptions on narcissistic transference are satisfactory.

Rosenfeld's own achievement was that he clarified the functioning of the defence mechanism, especially the relation to narcissism in negative therapeutic responses, by scrutinizing the object relationship in such narcissistic transferences. In addition, in contrast to previous researchers who studied narcissism mainly in schizophrenia —they were British researchers, and some American researchers—, Rosenfeld also studied much milder narcissistic patients including those who were socially successful.

He based his approaches on the Kleinian theory and was critical of Freud's view that primary narcissism was an objectless world and considered that it was in fact a primitive object relationship. He also stated that in such narcissistic object relationship, mainly two defence mechanisms, that is, omnipotence and identification with the object, are active.

Through omnipotence, the mother's breast or the care of the mother, as a part object, is omnipotently incorporated and becomes the babies' own property. Babies omnipotently project a part of their undesired self into the object. Furthermore, through projection/incorporation, the incorporated object and the self identifies and the boundary with the object disappears. Projective identification also causes a highly active movement in which a part of the self enters the object and acquires the good parts of the object.

Rosenfeld believed that such a narcissistic object relationship was in fact a defence against separation from the object. If you become aware of the separation from the object, a sense of dependence on the object occurs, and anxiety is aroused, therefore, a narcissistic object relationship is a defence method to deny the separation itself. To acknowledge that you are dependent on the object means that you recognize your love for the object or the value of the object. If you recognize such things, it means you will accept the separation. Thus, frustration will occur in the end and emotions such as anxiety, pain and aggression arise. Rosenfeld proposed that we adopt such a narcissistic defence mechanism to defend such emotions.

In addition, when a good thing in the object is recognized, envy occurs, which the patient considers unbearable. An omnipotent narcissistic object relationship is a means of eliminating them. If objects are omnipotently possessed, neither envy nor frustration will occur.

Rosenfeld considered that the intensity of persistence of such omnipotent narcissistic object relationship was associated with the intensity of the patient's envy. Envy is a keyword for the Kleinians, and Rosenfeld uses it often —the meaning of envy is the impulse to destroy what is good for oneself. He also focuses on the point where patients immediately exclude their undesirable things from the therapist, depreciate the therapist and use the object like a toilet without showing any compassion at all.

The above basic narcissistic object relationships are clinically expressed in various ways depending on the pathological condition. In extremely severe cases, the defence is obstinate and strongly defends the psychic reality. The patients lock themselves in a narcissistic world and try to exclude all conflicts. The defended anxiety in such cases is paranoic. An amazingly ideal conflict-free object relationship is developed there. Objects used like toilets are also idealized, and patients consider themselves as ideal beings, being loved by everything, and possessing all the good things. All therapeutic interventions that interfere with such state are strongly defended. Rosenfeld described a case patient who developed a typical narcissistic transference without becoming exceedingly psychotic.

Based on his experience with such cases, he found that clinically omnipotent and superior attitudes acted as rigid resistance and described the type of patients called intelligent narcissists who completely refuse to accept the value of the analyst. They take all the interpretations given to them by the therapist as if they were their own understanding and extract the meaning of the interpretations or develop the theory themselves. By doing so, patients maintain their ideal self-image and impede the analysis to develop.

Rosenfeld said that the prognosis of such patients depended on to what degree the patients could acknowledge their relationship with the analyst and that some patients whose degree of narcissism was not so strong and who had a part of self which was oriented to more normal objects could integrate with it.

The following paper was written in 1971 and describes "A Clinical Approach to the Psychoanalytic Theory of the Life and Death Instincts: An Investigation into the Aggressive Aspects of Narcissism", and additionally considers the characteristics of narcissism, especially the destructive aspect. A person of narcissism is a type of person who develops a negative treatment reaction in treatment and causes various problems such as interrupting the treatment in the middle or showing suicidal behaviour. Rosenfeld gives a deeper consideration on the destructive aspects of such narcissism by referring to Freud's idea of death instinct and Klein's idea of envy.

Rosenfeld believed that Freud did not give a consideration on the relationship between narcissistic withdrawal and "death instinct" even though he had clearly noticed it, and that Freud did not think that the negative treatment responses had anything to do with the narcissistic state although he had considered that it had a relationship with the death instinct. Rosenfeld considered that Klein's study on the "paranoid-schizoid position" contributed most to the study of narcissism. Klein's "paranoid-schizoid position" is well known in Japan, too. Rosenfeld referred to Klein's idea that life and death instincts are distributed in the process where individuals split off the self and the object.

Kleinians often use the words "life and death instinct", or envy, however, this has caused controversy. I, the author, also cannot agree with the idea that it is endogenous. However, what is clinically important is that the Kleinians proposed that envy was a conflict of the two dispositions, aggression and "life instinct" —a good disposition such as love for the object.

Rosenfeld considered that the sexual aspect of narcissism is related to overestimating and idealizing the self. By doing so, individuals omnipotently incorporate the good objects of the outside world and can feel that everything belongs to themselves and is under their control. On the other hand, in the destructive aspect of narcissism, where self-idealization plays an important role, the omnipotent and destructive part of self is idealized there. As a result, it destroys such things as the dependent good object relationship and the self's desire for the object. It is considered that this is related to the fact that narcissistic individuals are indifferent to the outside world.

Rosenfeld thought that the narcissism of most patients exhibits these two characteristics although the degree varies. In clinical practice, when the sexual aspect of narcissism is dominant, the patient assumes that the good aspect of the external object is his/hers, however, when the omnipotent self-idealization is threatened by transference interpretation, the underlying destructiveness is revealed, and the patient begins to notice his/her envy.

On the contrary, when the destructive aspect is dominant, the envy is more violent, and the patient thinks he/she wants to destroy the analyst and begins to possess a self-destructive impulse. In such cases, the patient feels that he/she would rather die than realize that he/she is dependent on the analyst or try to stop the treatment by disrupting the therapeutic progress or insight. In addition, the patient ruins his/her own professional life, or develops suicide wishes, suicide attempts, death wishes, idealization of death, or a situation where the patient forgets everything. At this time, the patient's entire self appears to be completely identified with the destructive part of self which is filled with envy. The patient destroys his/her own sexual self and demolishes his/her ability to care for others and his/her love. When this problem is treated well in treatment, behaviours such as compassion for the therapist appears.

However, in some patients, such destructive impulse is permanently ingrained into their entire personality and begins to affect the object relation. The sexual self of such patients is almost inactive, and they remove most of their power to love and care for others. They come to devote themselves to depreciating and becoming disinterested in or punishing the therapist and they become exultantly triumphant about losing objects.

In this way, when the whole self is identified with the part of the destructive narcissistic self, some often become organized. Rosenfeld says this can be compared to something like a gang led by a leader, just like a criminal organization. The purpose of such a systematic defence organization is to maintain the status quo and eliminate the benign self. Receiving help or undergoing change means his/her weakness and the patient cannot stand it. Therefore, the patient strongly resists the treatment. According to Rosenfeld, there is a perverted fusion of "life and death instinct" here, and the patient has turned the aggressive impulse into a kind of pleasure and has fallen into a perverted object relation.

Rosenfeld described the relationship between narcissism and negative treatment responses, the relationship between destructive narcissism and death instinct, and its relationship to treatment impasse, in the third chapter of the book "Impasse and Interpretation", which was published in 1987 after his death. The basic idea is presented in the two papers mentioned above. Another psychoanalyst called Leslie Sohn also studied narcissism, however, the details will be omitted here.

What I would like to add is that the idea that there exists a bad self which overwhelmingly dominates the other good parts of the self, such like a gang, is the core perspective of the present Kleinians. It is an idea called pathological organization which the self is distortedly identified with. Research is actively being conducted to make use of this to understand severe patients, including patients with perversion or addiction, borderline cases, narcissistic patients, and psychotic patients.

Next, I would like to briefly describe one of my own cases. It is a patient who very clearly expressed Rosenfeld's narcissistic defence.

The patient, Ms. A was an unmarried woman in her forties who came to see the therapist twice a week for about two and a half years and her chief complaint was sexual frigidity. She had been dating her boyfriend for about 5 years, but she came to see me with a chief complaint that she did not have any sexual pleasure at all. She was a clerk and the eldest of three siblings.

Her father did not have a regular job and had several part-time jobs such as a parttime teacher. He had a slightly eccentric personality, was selfish, and exploded his emotions with trifle things and her mother was always obedient. Only the patient confronted her father, and the other siblings immediately locked themselves up in their rooms when he had a tantrum. When she was 12 years old, she finally had a huge fight with her father. She said that she thought she won and had not talked with him properly ever since.

According to the patient, her mother was a truly kind passive person who worked and was often not at home for night shifts when the patient was small.

Patient Ms. A was dating Mr. B who was a divorced man some years older than her, when treatment started. Mr. B was very keen on her, but the patient had been dating him for about five years saying she did not know if she really loved him.

There is a characteristic in Ms. A's relationship with Mr. B. She set a condition on him that they will not interfere with each other's lives. Ms. A has several boyfriends and had dates with them every day alternately. She got sexual satisfaction when she sometimes had sexual intercourses with them. However, it just did not work with Mr. B. Even when Mr. B met another woman or his ex-wife, she pretended that she did not care. I only took up episodes, but when I pointed out in the therapeutic situation that Ms. A was actually feeling jealous or lonely about such things, she strongly denied it. After the sessions ended, she would say things like "I have a date with another boyfriend," or allude that she might have a sexual relationship.

When I, the therapist, pointed out that Ms. A was trying to consider that I was just one of those male followers and deny that she was in need of treatment, she would just laugh and refuse to deal with my interpretation. She also said that she had so many boyfriends and that even though she did not have any feelings for them, they desired her, and even if one or two of them left her, it was okay because there would be a next.

When Ms. A told me such things, I gave interpretations such as that, by doing so, she could quickly switch to the next boyfriend no matter whom she broke up with and was trying to avoid the pain of breaking up. I continued that she was denying all her parts which want to rely on people and desire people, and instead projecting those feelings into these boyfriends and despising them, trying to control her feelings, and have control over her boyfriends. However, Ms. A just listened silently.

In the meantime, Mr. B could not stand it anymore and began to say that he would work in another city as a seasonal worker for a while. Ms. A came to me and lied that Mr. B could go if he wanted to, and that she had plenty more alternative boyfriends. The therapist repeatedly interpreted that the patient actually did not want to lose him and did not want him to go but the feelings of separation were so painful that she was denying them all.

As I repeatedly gave interpretations, Ms. A gradually became aware of her feelings, and at the farewell party, she got dead drunk and clung to Mr. B in tears saying, "Don't go," and made a show of herself. Thereafter, Ms. A came to treatment and blamed the therapist in extreme vexation saying that it was not her intention to play such a blunder, and she was just influenced by the suggestion of the therapist.

When Mr. B actually went to another city, Ms. A started dating another boyfriend from the very day. When she came to the treatment, she said that Mr. B, who had gone away, became a past person in a few days, and that she had forgotten him. Even when the therapist once and again pointed out that that was the way to somehow manage her pain of abandonment anxiety, she gave no clear answer.

Two weeks later, Mr. B contacted Ms. A and told her that he had become ill and was hospitalized in another city and that he wanted to come back to her home town after he got well. Ms. A said to me, "I've forgotten Mr. B and have started a new free life, so it's such a nuisance." When the therapist interpreted that, by doing so, Ms. A was trying to get her revenge on Mr. B, who abandoned her, she just kept silent and listened.

Mr. B came back and took a rest for a while in Ms. A's apartment, but she looked down on him, saying that she was disappointed with him because he was leaning on her and looked weak. However, Mr. B became well aware that he needed her after going to another and asked her to marry him. At that moment, Ms. A thought that she had won, and her spirits lifted. She despised the pitiful Mr. B, and replied, "I don't know if I will." However, she would not break up with him.

The therapist pointed out that the patient was disdainful of her own feeling that desires people, so when she saw it in a person, she despised that person. However, the patient did not answer anything and just listened. The patient showed various different attitudes; she sometimes listened with a serious look, and sometimes with an incredibly scornful look.

What was notable during this period was that Ms. A began to call her mother and return home on weekends. Ms. A never did so until then. She would not go home even on Christmas Eve, but she began to return every week. She would go home and talk with her mother and siblings. Furthermore, she and her sibling who was in the same city as her started to stay at each other's place. I thought this indicated that although the patient had a narcissistic defence mechanism, on the other hand, her sexual desire to the object was growing.

What I also focused on was that Ms. A, who was from a place far away from the city she lived in, accepted her father to stay at her apartment when he came to her city and asked her if she would let him stay. She had obstinately refused until then. She started talking with her father, too, little by little.

In the meantime, Ms. A began to realize that she could not separate with Mr. B and accepted his proposal. However, she did not make clear when they would get married. She promised that she would marry him after they had found a place to live, and they started looking for a house. This was an incredibly symbolic event which indicated that the patient expressed her intention to share a common world with the object. However, this house-hunting took an awful lot of time. She did not like any of the houses she went and saw. She viewed dozens of houses for more than half a year, however, there was always some point she did not like, so they were having a hard time to get settled.

Ms. A's relationship with Mr. B was still unsteady, and she sometimes dated other boyfriends. In such a situation, Mr. B suggested going on a trip, but at the destination, Ms. A obstinately refused to have sex. Mr. B got angry and did things such as introduce another girlfriend to her. The patient insisted to the therapist, "I don't care about that, I have many other boyfriends." Even when the therapist pointed out that Ms. A was actually angry at Mr. B and was jealous of the woman, she refused to accept.

Then, Ms. A suddenly decided to change her workplace to a small town which took two hours from the city she used to live in. The therapist said it was apparent that she did so to run away from her feelings and protest against Mr. B because she was angry with him and suffered from jealousy, but she would not listen. She thus decided to drive two hours each way, twice a week, to come to me for treatment.

However, once she began to work at her new workplace, Ms. A felt that it did not suit her on the very first day and returned to her former workplace in the previous city she lived in even though she had to pay compensation for the breach of contract. The therapist repeatedly pointed out to her that it was apparent that she did so because she felt that she needed Mr. B but did not want to notice, and would feel jealousy and have a painful experience of being abandoned if she acknowledged her feelings. This made the patient extremely angry with the therapist, and she left the room in the middle of the session saying that the therapist's words were no help for her, and they were incomprehensible.

Here is another episode: The patient was 45 minutes late because of snow for the first session after the discontinuation of treatment because the therapist took a winter vacation for two weeks. She rushed into the interview room breathlessly. There were only 5 minutes left because the next patient was waiting then. As soon as Ms. A entered the room and met the therapist, she suddenly noticed that she had bothered to endure the traffic jam and come all the way to meet the therapist and made a downright vexatious look. Consciously for her, the therapist was just one of her many men followers, and had been an object that could be replaced any time, however, now that she had come to realize that she needed the therapist, she thought it was extremely vexing.

In such way, Ms. A lived in an omnipotent narcissistic world where she completely denied that she needed the objects and projected her dependency onto the objects. She thought she was loved by all the men around her and they were under her control. Although she would not clearly affirm with words that she directly accepted the importance of the relationship with the therapist, as the therapist interpreted her narcissistic defence mechanism at every opportunity, she began to meet her mother and family.

As I mentioned earlier, this patient came to treatment about twice a week for two years and three months with almost no cancellations. In the meantime, she got another boyfriend —a person who listened especially to her and understood everything— and had long talks with him regularly every week. The therapist interpreted this as a clear representation of a part of a positive transference. Although the patient would just nod and not affirm clearly, I felt she understood. It is considered that the sadomasochistic relationship with her father is clearly related to the formation of such an object relation, and that the fact that the mother who should have satisfied her desire was often absent is also related to it.

In addition, her other various episodes tell that Ms. A was a person who often had traumatic experiences. The defence mechanism she took at that time was probably identification with her father's awfully aggressive attitude to try to deal with her painful experience.

Technically, I concentrated on interpreting the patient's separation experience caused by narcissistic defence consisting of what Rosenfeld described, e.g., omnipotence, projection, introjection, and projective identification, and interpreting the defence against traumatic experiences. Practically, when I felt that the patient was denying things such as the patient's desire for the object, her dependency or her experience when losing the object, I tried to use confrontation.

While I attended her with such an approach, the patient's sexual feeling, in other words, her desire for the object, gradually became stronger, and eventually Ms. A said that she would finally marry her original boyfriend, Mr. B. Around that time, my treatment came to an end.

Note: This paper is a revised version of the presentation record of an Educational Seminar.

References

(1) Abraham, Karl. 1919/1927. "A Particular Form of Neurotic Resistance Against the Psychoanalytic Method". In *Selected Papers of Karl Abraham*: 301-311. London: Hogarth Press.

(2) Freud, Sigmund. 1914. "On Narcissism: An Introduction". In *Standard Edition*, Vol 14: 67-102. London: Hogarth Press.

(3) Reich, Wilhelm. 1933. *Character Analysis*. New York: Orgone Institute Press.

(4) Rosenfeld, Herbert. 1964/1965. "On the Psychopathology of Narcissism: A Clinical Approach". In *Psychotic States*. London: Hogarth Press.

(5) Rosenfeld, Herbert. 1971. "A Clinical Approach to the Psychoanalytic Theory of the Life and Death Instincts: An Investigation into the Aggressive Aspects of Narcissism". *International Journal of Psychoanalysis*, Vol. 52: 169-178.

(6) Rosenfeld, Herbert. 1987. *Impasse and Interpretation*. New York and London: Tavistock.

(7) Sohn, Louis. 1985/1988. "Narcissistic Organization, Projective Identification and the Formation of the Identificate". *International Journal of Psychoanalysis*, Vol. 66: 201- 213; reprinted in *Melanie Klein Today*, Vol. 1. edited by Elizabeth Spillius, 324-342. London: Routledge.

(8) Steiner. John. 1993. *Psychic Retreats.* London: Routledge.

[1992. *The Japanese Journal of Psycho-analysis*, Vol. 35, No. 5.]

CHAPTER 2

THE MOURNING WORK AND ITS PATHOLOGICAL STATE

1. Introduction

The concept of mourning work was clarified by Freud in a paper entitled "Mourning and Melancholia" (1917) [2], and since then it has been considered as the most important developmental emotional experience in the studies of psychoanalysis and developmental psychology. Basic research on it also has greatly progressed as a study of the infant's separation experience from the mother, owing to analysts including Bowlby [1] in the United Kingdom and Mahler [6] et al. in the United States. Furthermore, along with the development of psychosomatic medicine, the issue of object loss has attracted attention in the study of stress and psychosomatic correlation. In other words, in stress evaluation questionnaires, it has become clear that the experience of object loss, such as loss of a spouse, is one of the items that show the largest stress coefficient. Moreover, object loss and mourning work have come to gain attention from researchers in a wide range of fields [7], [8].

Mourning work refers to the entire psychological process in which an individual gradually recovers from the grief associated with the experience of object loss. Loss experience includes many experience worlds in daily life as follows: 1) separation from or bereavement of a close person such as a family member, 2) experience of losing material things such as property, 3) loss of social self-image such as failure of promotion or work, 4) developmentally inevitable loss as a person grows (e.g., independence from parents in adolescence, retirement, death of spouse or oneself due to aging), and 5) loss of physical function or physical self-image, and loss of social self-image, etc. due to illness or handicap. A healthy person can successfully carry out mourning work, and can gradually accept the real world in which he/she has lost his/her object, and eventually start a new life. However, some people are unable to carry out a healthy mourning work, and develop pathological symptoms such as depression, psychotic conditions, and neurosis as a result of the loss experience [(3), (7), (8)].

There are many possible factors that determine the course of this mourning work, but generally they include the followings [(3)]: (1) The value and symbolic meaning of the loss for the individual: The loss can be many things, such as parents, property, or physical function, and there are many kinds of variations in loss experiences. Especially in the case of individuals who have lost their parents, ambivalent relationships with them while they were alive are considered to have a significant impact on mourning work. (2) The age of the individual when he/she had the loss experience: For example, even in the experience of losing a mother, it is natural that the ego's processing ability, semantic experience and other matters are different in the case of infants, adolescents, and adults. In the former two cases, it may leave a significant influence on personality formation and formation of predispositions such as mental illness. (3) Individual personality before the loss experience: This also has a great relation to the individual ego's coping ability for mourning work. (4) Supporting and coping ability of close relatives such as family members. (5) Supporting and accepting ability of medical personnel and society: Various factors are involved, particularly, the issue of social acceptance and rejection of handicaps. Each individual will follow a unique process of mourning work.

2. Case

Here, I would like to report a patient who failed to go through such mourning work and presented pathological conditions, and describe the influence on her mental health. This case patient presented chronic neurotic symptoms triggered by the death of a family member (her father), which is the most typical loss experience.

Patient

The patient was a 28-year-old unmarried woman. She was an aspiring actor and made her living while working as a secretary.

Current medical history and life history

She had continued to have chronic compulsive behaviour since her father died when the patient was 8 years old. For example, the patient had fear that her mother would die if the patient did not blink 8 times at the moment a car passed by, and had a magical thinking that her father would come back to life if she hit a nearby object multiple times. Furthermore, when she became an adult, she had to make sure that all the bar lock handles in the room were turned up and that they were locked properly. Since she repeated this no matter what kind of sociable situation she went to, social life became difficult and it had an injurious influence on her relationships with people around her.

She had had chronic depression and suicidal ideation since her junior high school days, but said she could not commit suicide when she thought of her mother. The patient hated herself and suffered from inferiority complex, and tended to feel guilty about everything. Since the death of her father, the patient had never felt happy. She suffered from a sense of isolation, and felt that she was wasting her life without anything to live for. The degree of these chronic depressive states changed slightly as the patient grew, however, they did not improve.

Physically, she also had continued to have symptoms including headaches, haemorrhoid, chronic gastritis, and enlarged tonsils for a long time since her father died when she was 8 years old.

At the diagnostic interview, the patient was very particular about death. She described that many people around her had died. The first death was the death of her father when she was 8 years old. After her father died, the patient and her family began to live with her grandparents, who died when the patient was 16 and 20 years old, respectively. When the patient was 24 years old, her paternal aunt, whom she admired, died. This aunt lived in the patient's neighbourhood and she took good care of the patient. In addition, when the patient was 12 years old, her neighbour classmate friend was killed in a plane accident. The patient said those many deaths had devastated her.

The patient has kept on studying although she has been suffering from compulsive behaviour and depression since she was 8 years old. She visited a child psychiatrist at the age of 9 and received outpatient treatment for 3 months. At that time, although she did not get completely better, the degree of obsessive-compulsive symptoms was slightly reduced, so she stopped going to the hospital. In her junior high school days, compulsive behaviour and the depressive state became stronger, but she managed to continue going to school without seeing a psychiatrist. Although she suffered from symptoms and continued to have a lonely high school life, she kept on studying diligently and her school grades were good. She proceeded to the department of English language and literature of a university and achieved excellent grades. She then entered an acting school with the aim of becoming an actor and graduated in three years. In this manner, obsessive-compulsive symptoms and depressive states did not completely suppress the patient's basic social life, despite they prolonged for a long time and imposed considerable restrictions on her life. However, before she came to my clinic, the above symptoms worsened due to troubles with her boyfriend and isolation among her peer actors, thus the patient herself decided to receive psychoanalytic psychotherapy and came for consultation.

Family members

- Father

He was a company worker and was healthy. He died of acute heart failure during sleep (35 years old) when the patient was 8 years old. The patient said that she was his favourite and she liked him more than she liked her mother. The night before her father suddenly died, the patient did something wrong and was scolded by her mother, and she did not listen to her father even when he told her to, so he did not give her his usual good-night kiss. Her father suddenly died without reconciling with her so it has become a strong guilty feeling for the patient.

- Mother

She was 52 years old. According to the patient, her mother was dominant and self-centred. After her husband's death, she worked as a hairdresser to sustain the household, but she remarried two years later. The mother was dependent on the patient, but on the other hand, she tried to control everything about the patient. The patient also established a dependent relationship with her mother after her father's death and tried to follow her mother's opinion in everything. However, she had hatred and anger against her self-centred and dominant mother. Nevertheless, the patient needed experience of self-exploration with psychotherapy to be clearly aware of this. In other words, before the death of her father, the patient hated her dominant mother and had a strong attachment to her father. However, after the death of her father, the only person the patient could rely on was her mother. According to the patient, the patient cried to and leant on her mother like a baby. At the diagnostic interview, the patient's mind was so preoccupied with the thought that her mother would also die if the patient did not perform a compulsive ritual, she could not realize her hostility against her mother.

- Brother

He was 32 years old. Like the patient, the sudden death of their father had become a major traumatic experience for him. The relationship with his mother had not worked well and he tended to be a rebellious, domestically violent, self-destructive man.

- Father-in-law

He was 54 years old. When the patient was 10 years old, he remarried her mother. His ex-wife died when she gave birth to their younger daughter. When he remarried, the child was 10 months old. The patient was hardly attached to him and their relationship was tenuous.

- Sisters-in-law

They were 28 and 19 years old, respectively. Their relationships with the patient were shallow. As a child, the patient had a stormy relationship with her two sisters-in-law. Her older sister-in-law also suffered from depressive neurotic symptoms.

As described above, the case patient was a patient who had a traumatic loss experience, and had hardly overcome that experience through mourning work. Therefore, she was chronically suffering from pathological obsessive-compulsive symptoms, depressive states, and physical symptoms. In addition, her mother had also failed to achieve mourning work for that loss experience, and had become dependent on the patient. The mother had continued to have an interdependent and integrated relationship with the patient. As a result, the mother could not sympathize with the desperate world of the patient's loss experience. Instead, the patient was forced to take mental care of her mother.

The man whom the mother remarried had just lost his wife. This entire stepfamily tried to use each other to fill in their experiences of object loss, leaving each one unable to carry out mourning work successfully. The patient's brother and older sister-in-law also had neurotic problems.

3. Therapeutic course

In the early stages of treatment, the patient's pathology was clearly manifested in the transference relation and free associations that the patient developed. They clearly indicated that the mourning work for the death of her father had failed. The patient was treated by psychoanalytic therapy 3 times a week, and after 2 years of treatment, the symptoms disappeared and interpersonal relationships improved, so the treatment was terminated.

At the start of treatment, the patient was in an extremely anxious and desperate state. She talked rapidly on and on about the details of the many deaths in addition to her father's death. She often asked if the male therapist would understand and help her with them.

In addition, the patient reported many dreams from the beginning of therapy, most of which were about death. For example, "I became very jealous when my boyfriend was with another woman. The boyfriend died.

My mother was by my side and he came back to life.", "My father-in-law and mother got divorced. My dead father appears and becomes arrogant and takes my mother away. And I am left alone.", and "My birth father is hospitalized for a serious illness, and his whole body is dirty with stool and urine. I sang a song and washed them off with shampoo." In those dreams, there was a world of magical desires where her father was not yet dead in her mind or where she tried to bring him back to life. They expressed that she was still suffering from ambivalent feelings towards her dead father.

She also said that the men she dated kept on leaving her, and repeatedly said that she needed them even though she did not love them. Such object relations with men were repeatedly seen with 2 or 3 men. This also was considered to represent the influence of the ambivalent relationship with the inner representation of her father, who suddenly left her behind. This disposition was clearly demonstrated in the transference to the therapist. That is, once she met the therapist, she became dependent on him, although he was supposed to be an unimportant man for the patient. She worried that the therapist might leave her someday, or the therapist would die during the vacation, and she would be hurt again.

Regarding her mother, the patient kept on crying showing her strong anxiety: "My father and men have left me, but only my mother does not leave me. I hate my mother because she suffocates me, but I absolutely need such a mother." and "I had vaguely realized that I hated my mother because she was dominant, but if I'm not a good girl, I would hurt her and she also might die." At one point, the patient asked her mother on the phone, "What will you do if I marry a non-Jewish man or kill a person?" (The patient was Jewish.) The patient said in tears, "My mother said she would still accept me, so I'm sorry for my mother." This expressed her separation anxiety and how strong her sense of guilt was when she did not follow her mother's intension. In addition, the patient said, "I'm like being connected to my mother by an umbilical cord, and only my mother accepts me. I want to see her. I want to be a baby and disappear in her arms. But I want to be independent, I want to be a person who doesn't need her." She poured out an extremely ambivalent disposition against her mother, which was originally related to her father's death.

Such stories were also linked to the transference relationship with the therapist. For example, when separation with the therapist became a problem because there were no treatment sessions for a while due to vacation, the patient would cry intensely remembering the scene where she saw her mother off at the station when her mother had to go to another city for hair dressing training 2 weeks after her father's death. She said, "I need my mother. I want to be a baby and go back into her womb. But I don't want to rely on my completely controlling mother. I have to be independent." The patient also developed this ambivalent relationship with the therapist. The patient did not bring a watch. She hated being told the treatment time, and disliked leaving the room. Then again, the patient came to complain that the therapist's room was like a prison, and that if she was locked in once, she would not be able to leave the room. There was something common to the relationship with her mother. In regard to this, the therapist pointed out to the patient that, in the back of her mind, she was experiencing the ambivalence of the same quality as the feelings for her mother in the separation from the therapist during the vacation. The patient denied, but it seemed she did so because she would recall her painful emotions if she became aware of the ambivalence. The patient disliked hearing the therapist's interpretations and sometimes rejected them angrily, but her subsequent associations showed that such interventions were correct.

The patient could not share her loss experience with her mother, but instead took care of her mother. She became a good girl, and sacrificed herself to repair her mother's apparently unsuccessful loss experience. Instead, she continued long to be in a state where she relieved her anxiety of isolation by clinging on to her mother. This was a form of "false self". Mourning work on the death of the patient's father seemed to have never been completed between the two of them.

4. Consideration

In this way, the pathology caused by the failure of mourning work for the sudden death of the patient's father was clearly demonstrated in the early treatment associations and transference relationship. The patient still possessed a living father in her mind; the father was not dead in the patient's unconsciousness. The patient had tried to deny the reality of her father's death for nearly 20 years. The mother also had hardly completed mourning work, and she had not been able to assist the patient's mourning work. The patient had made efforts to somehow cope with the experience of her father's sudden death by having a symbiotic relationship with such mother. There was no sympathy that promoted each other's mourning work, and they had been supporting each other in a way that rejected it. The mother's remarriage to a man who had just lost his wife may have further strengthened this.

As can be clearly seen in the transference, for the patient, men were existences that abandoned her and disappeared, and existences that died when she depended on them. On the other hand, although women did not resolve the patient's suffering of death separation, they were objects who survived, whom the patient could depend on. Especially, her mother was the only object of dependency who protected the patient from isolation. Such patient tried to avoid separating from her mother even by sacrificing her self. However, when she was near by her mother, the patient felt suffocated and her hatred being dominated by her mother enhanced. Nevertheless, if the patient departed from her mother, the patient was unable to deal with the problem of her father's death and her lonely world where she was isolated from her mother. One of the methods the patient adopted was to throw herself, who sought for an object that would heal her, into her mother through the mechanism of projective identification, and handle herself by taking care of her mother.

Freud [(2)] studied the disposition where individuals tried to solve such psychology of object loss by introjecting the lost parents (external objects) into their minds, identifying with them, and becoming like the lost persons. Klein [(4), (5)] established a theory that focused on the object relation between the internal "good object" and "bad object" based on the concept of the "depressive position". When individuals lose a family member or the like, they lose not only an external object but also an internal object. For example, if a father dies suddenly, the individual loses not only the external father but also the internal father. At this point, when the ambivalence between hatred and affection in the previous relation with the lost object was strong, the negative feelings of being left behind are intense and it will take time to restore the lost object as a good object. Furthermore, the individual cannot utilize external assistance well, and he/she will not be able to carry out mourning work successfully.

Furthermore, in a case where the experience is too traumatic, even if the relationship with the lost object had been relatively good, if external assistance is not appropriate, the ego cannot complete mourning work, thus, cannot recover the lost good internal object. Especially when the individual is a child, such as the case patient, appropriate support and understanding from the surrounding people such as the mother are important factors for successful mourning work. In that respect, the coping ability of the subject, such as the age of the individual when he/she had the experience of object loss, and the environmental conditions are also major factors for mourning work to succeed.

In the case of this patient, the relationship with her lost father was relatively favourable, but the child's ego did not have enough capability to complete mourning work. In addition, it must have been difficult for the mother to assist the patient's mourning work in situations where the patient-mother relationship was ambivalent and the mother herself had not successfully overcome mourning work for the loss experience of her husband's death.

5. Conclusion

As a specific case of mourning work pathology, I introduced and added consideration on a case patient who continued to have compulsive behaviour, depression, and physical symptoms for a long period of 20 years because her father died of heart failure during sleep when the patient was 8 years old. I also showed that the symbiotic relationship with the remaining mother further prevented the mourning work, and that the pathology of object loss was clearly expressed in the therapeutic relationship. I further introduced the studies of Freud and Klein on object loss and the mourning work.

References

(1) Bowlby, John. 1969/1973. *Attachment and Loss*, Vol. 1-2. New York: Basic Books.

(2) Freud, Sigmund. 1917. "Mourning and Melancholia". In *Standard Edition of the Complete Psychological Works of Sigmund Freud*, Vol.14, 243-258. London: Hogarth Press.

(3) Kinugasa, Takayuki. 1980. "Psychological Features and Psychotherapeutic Problems of Patients with Physical Handicaps". *The Japanese Journal of Psycho-analysis*, Vol. 25, No.2: 69-77 (in Japanese)

(4) Klein, Melanie. 1935. "A contribution to the Psychogenesis of Manic-Depressive States". *International Journal of Psychoanalysis,* Vol. 16: 145-174.

(5) Klein, Melanie. 1940/1975. "Mourning and Its Relation to Manic-Depressive States". In *The Writings of Melanie Klein*, Vol. 1, 344-269. London: Hogarth Press.

(6) Mahler, Margaret S., Pine, Fred, and Bergman, Anni. 1975. *The Psychological Birth of the Human Infant*. New York: Basic Books.

(7) Okonogi, Keigo. 1979. *Object Loss – To Mourn*. Tokyo: Chuokoron-Shinsha. (in Japanese)

(8) Okonogi, Keigo. 1991. "Object Loss and Mourning Work". *The Japanese Journal of Psycho-analysis*, Vol. 34, No. 5: 294-322 (in Japanese)

[1994. *The Japanese Journal of Stress Sciences*, Vol. 3, No. 3.]

CHAPTER 3

ON THE FORMATION OF THE BODY IMAGES IN PSYCHOSIS: IN KLEINIAN THOUGHTS

1. Introduction

When we recognize others, we cannot capture them without their body images, especially their facial expressions which are a special part of the body. The existence of the body is the basis of an individual, however, on the other hand, we intuitively understand and face that other people have a mind inside their body. Moreover, we cannot think about our self without our physical presence, and we also intuitively grasp that our mind exists somewhere inside that body. Although it is considered that this is already functioning in infants and children, there are still many unknown parts about the generation process.

Some psychotic patients exhibit phenomena where they feel that their mind exists outside the body, or feel that there are souls which do not have a body, and there are a group of patients whose body images themselves are considered mentally ill such as patients with hypochondria and psychosomatic disorders. In order to understand such people, it is important to understand how the body self-image and the object image are generated. However, at the present stage, it is difficult to say that this theme is sufficiently studied.

Originally in psychoanalysis, body-centred drive theory, anxiety generation theory and object relation theory have been developed and the body plays an important role, however, it is difficult to say that its mental function and the problem of the body self have been clarified. S. Freud developed the instinct theory which aims to satisfy the instinctive pleasures of the maturity of the body and openings of the body in a developmental theory based on drive theory.

Some researchers such as P. Schilder and E. Bick consider that physical contact when the mother takes care of the baby greatly influences the formation of the baby's body self, and pay attention to the existence of skin as the boundary between the inside and outside of self. Furthermore, the

Kleinian concept of phantasy activities related to the inside of the body has a potential to make an important contribution in the study of body image formation. Although psychoanalysts including M. Klein do not actively take up the problem of the body image of self, they consider that part object phantasies and the whole object image in the integration of them as something that can be grasped physically, and have made many highly suggestive references.

2. Klein's study on body phantasy

Klein explained the early object relation with the concepts of paranoid-schizoid position and depressive position. In "Psychoanalysis of Children", all the states of activity of early object relation are described as exchanges between the object body and the self body. The overview is summarized in the abstract of the academic conference so it will be omitted here. The activities of early object relation, which occur in the pre-verbal world, are complex activities of the internal world, which are experienced as activities of phantasy. It is a world of concrete phantasy, and a world where object representation and abstract thinking are not fully developed yet. In infants and children, it is often difficult to distinguish phantasies from external reality. The babies' world of internal phantasy is also considered to be almost equivalent to the actual experience. In any case, it is exceedingly difficult to capture what the mental activity of this period is like. The activity of the children's phantasies differs from adults' fantasy and imagination activities and they are the basic materials which form the core of the self and the objects themselves. It is considered that sensory impressions such as visual sensory impression, auditory sensory impression and tactile sensory impression of the body play a big role in this. In the phantasy activity, the world of concrete exchanges between the partial body-others and body-self is active there. The worlds of others-body and self-body are gradually constructed, and the self fits into the body. Then a self which can examine the reality that others exist outside the skin and inside the others-body is established.

An integrated self-body image will come into existence at the time when the integrating stages develop after the depressive position, similarly to the formation of the others-body image.

In Klein's research, although the object's body phantasy is described in details, the infants' and children's own self-body phantasies and the phantasies inside their bodies are only mentioned briefly. From the subject side of infants and children, it seems relatively easy to grasp the mother's body object with senses such as visual, auditory, tactile, and gustatory senses in early object relations. In addition, babies can see their mother's expressions and body. However, babies cannot see their own expression and it is difficult for them to directly see their entire body. Spontaneously, infants gradually discover a part of their body sensation through actions such as finger sucking. Experiences of hunger, satisfaction, pain, pleasure, discomfort of wet diapers, pleasure and pain of defecation become the grounds of the inner body sensation. Skin sensation will be important to distinguish the inside and the outside of their body. It is something that is experienced through physical contact including cuddling by the mother's hands and arms in the care by the mother. Compared to the object's body image, the self body image of infants and children is something quite ambiguous which is formed while being largely influenced by emotions and drives. Actually, even for us adults, it is quite difficult to call up the body image of our own. As for their own body phantasies, infants are strongly influenced by their experiences with the objects and the phantasies of them. Many are formed through the reflection experiences with the objects and will be influenced by extremely subjective and emotional experiences. The bias of cathexis for the self body parts are greater compared to that for the object body image. In any case, as the object body phantasies are integrated, the subjective self-body phantasies associated with them will also be integrated. In this process, as described by Bick, the skin of self is thought to play an important role in distinguishing the inside from the outside. On the other hand, Klein and other psychoanalysts assume that the inside and the outside in part object relation exist from immediately after birth, and consider that splitting, projective identification and introjective identification occur from the beginning.

3. Bion's semiotic ontology and Bick's skin boundary theory

While considering the development and the formation process of psychotic and non-psychotic parts of personality, Bion tried to explain sense impressions, alpha-function, beta-elements, bizarre object, fragmentation, projective identification, and splitting with symbols such as L, H, and K. All of these are something that symbolize and conceptualize the states of various activities, mainly the functional aspect, such as projection and introjection of physical phantasies, in the process where part objects are integrated into whole objects. However, he focused on the formation of their mental function part and made a consideration on the process where thoughts, concepts, symbolization, and memories developed. Although he has not made much consideration on the body-self, he considered their actual mental activities as extremely physical part object or whole object phantasies.

Bick, who was strongly influenced by Bion, thought that the skin played an important role in differentiating the inside from the outside of self, as described above. Most of the care by the mother including lactation, cuddling, and dipper changing are conducted mainly through the skin sensation. This becomes the important sensation where the inside of the self and the inside of the body, and the outside of the body and what are not the self are distinguished around the border of the skin. Then, the babies introject the skin, which can be contained first, from the object. According to Bick, babies identify the firstly-introjected primary object with their skin, and thereby distinguish the outside from the inside. It is considered that babies then hold space within their body, keep what they introjected, and make it as the core of their self. This means the containing function of the primary object (the mother) is important. If this does not work well, it is considered that a defensive secondary skin is formed, and the problem of the world of autism which has no internal space is presented. The problem of psychogenic psychosomatic disorder may also lie in here.

As described above, Bick considered that the premise for conducting introjection from the object is established by the formation of an inner space in the self. Then, through the exchange where babies introject good objects into the skin self, and project and exclude the bad object world outside the skin body boundary, they form a steady world of self and objects.

4. Case Report — A male patient who expressed his body-self by drawing

I would like to present a case where a male patient who has suffered a psychotic breakdown depicted his self-image in his recovery process. Furthermore, I would like to show that the body-self is oddly distorted in the pathological condition of the paranoid/schizoid position. It is considered that the unresolved areas will be further elucidated by observing as many body images of patients with such psychotic problems as possible, and further accumulating early observation data of severe patients in infantile observation and psychoanalysis of children.

Case

The patient was a man in his 20s. His chief complaints were "My withdrawal has prolonged," "My soul will crush," "My words do not work," and "People's gazes make me feel uneasy."

Disease History and Diagnosis

Although the patient had experienced a transient psychotic state from about his junior high school days, he did not discontinue studying and his school achievements were good. He participated in a sports club without skipping until the third grade (the final grade) of high school. However, he tended to be interpersonally confined, and associated with people only superficially. He says that actually the door of his mind was kept closed. From the time he passed the university entrance examinations and started living in a boarding house away from his parents, the patient stayed in his room and did not go to university. His parents noticed this after sixth months from entrance and this is how the patient came for consultation. The diagnosis for him was severe schizoid disorder (psychotic personality).

Therapeutic Process

In the first year, the patient complained emotions such as a fear that his heart would crush if he used words and a fear that his heart would disappear, and often became silent during treatment. Even so, he gradually came to be able to talk about his family. He especially began to tell his anger and dissatisfaction against his parents and when the therapist's vacations and cancellations continued, he began to be silent for a long time and occasionally describe a destructive world. One day, the patient's parents stayed at his boarding house. His father kept on telling the patient subtle complaints and demands as usual. The patient's intense anger exploded against his father. From that time on, the patient developed symptoms including hallucination, delusional mood, and a feeling of persecution of being killed by someone, and the patient began to continuously shut himself up in his room. Although I recommended hospitalization, neither his family nor he himself agreed, therefore it was decided that he would continue to come to treatment while his mother took care of him at his boarding house. The patient would appear for psychotherapy on time without cancellations, however he kept silent, which continued for six months. The counter-transference experience during this time was like being in a strange hypnotic state for the therapist.

After the patient was in a psychotic condition for six months, one day, he broached that he wanted to do drawing and sculpture. Since silence accompanied by a prolonged psychotic state had continued, these words made me, the therapist, extremely happy; because I had waited and waited for clues of the patient's self-expression. From then on, the patient drew many pictures and made many pieces of work with clay. Many of them were composed of odd partial inconsistent things which seemed to depict the parts of his psychotic self. However, on the other hand, I, the therapist, considered that the function of his healthy ego which observed such psychotic parts and tried to tell them to me was beginning to come back into existence. I took the world of drawing and clay as a medium of the patient's primitive expression and communication. In addition, I determined my direction to understand the world of the meaning of those strange pictures and clay works by applying the techniques of dream analysis, and actively give interpretations when they expressed the patient's internal state or transferences. Here I would like to focus on the course of the six months when the patient started drawing and making clay works, and expressed his psychotic object images, state of ego and self-image, and also the depiction of his own self-image.

When the patient could think that the therapist's interpretations were right, he gave a small nod and subsequently continued with his creative drawing and clay work. At first, the patient drew pictures where various things and parts of the body with no lefts or rights, or tops or bottoms were fragmented and then assembled like a mosaic (**Picture 1**). The therapist asked for explanations on each of those parts, however the patients could not give explanations for many of them. Nevertheless, a drawing where a strange rocket was moving away from the earth (**Picture 2**) could be understood that it represented the separation experience when his mother's return to her hometown overlapped with the therapist's vacation. Furthermore, I gave interpretations for drawings such as the drawing of a transparent borderless vase with a flower whose leaves protruded from it (**Picture 3**) and the drawing of mechanical flowers grown in a greenhouse (**Picture 4**) because I considered they expressed the activity of the patient's internal mind. Concretely, I gave interpretations that, when the patient separated from the therapist, he experienced that he would go far away into the universe and would never be able to come back again, and that the patient experienced being maintained in treatment and felt flowers were beginning to gradually grow. After a while, the patient depicted a module in which something that seemed to be a person's face was multiply overlapped. It seemed to be his mother's face, and was probably one of his psychotic primitive object images (**Picture 5**). The patient made clay works at the same time for the first time then. He made an alcohol lamp first and changed it into a candle, a beer mug, a flower, and last into a Hamburg steak. While watching this, I interpreted that the patient "has gradually begun to feel that his world was being shed light on at the treatment site, and the patient was making a toast and expressing his joy with his favourite flower, and was achieving a sense of satisfaction as when he ate his favourite

Hamburg steak". Next, he drew an un-understandable fragmented picture, and made a neckless figure and a bottomless container with clay. This seemed to indicate that the patient did not want to understand the world interpreted by the therapist and could not retain it, either. In this way, the patient came to be able to express his mind brilliantly with drawing and clay work.

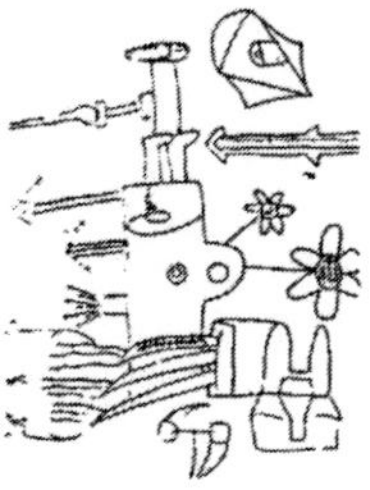

Picture 1

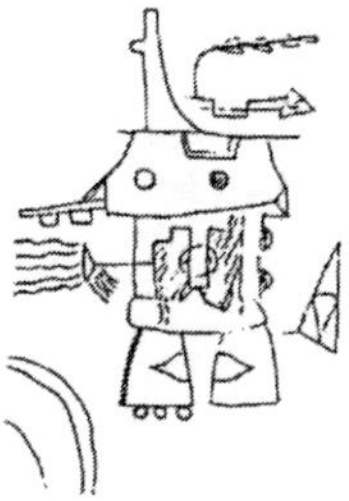

Picture 2

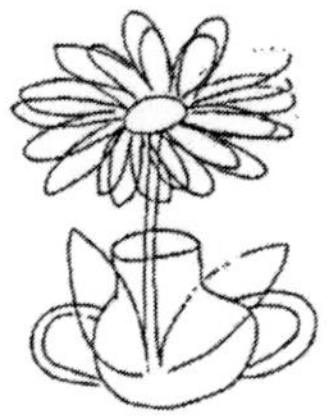

Picture 3

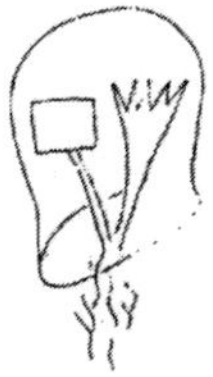

Picture 4

Before the following session, the patient's mother called and said in an angry tone, "My son touches my body and is all over me like a baby. When I am asleep, he will examine my mouth and eyes and rub his cheek against mine. He tries to touch my breasts and tummy, too. I think he is seriously ill and will not recover anymore." She then directly went back to her hometown. In the subsequent session, the patient made a flower that had fallen to the ground with clay, and drew a patchy picture of rain and clouds, a wind-blown tent, and a bird (often representing a handless self-image) and a heart (**Picture 6**). While listening to the patient's brief explanations, the therapist felt that he could understand what they were representing. I interpreted, "It is related to my vacation, and it expresses your bitterness and how you experienced a painful heart when your mother left." The patient nodded and confessed that his mother became angry because he had become childish like a kindergartener, and was trying to be all over her. He looked down.

In the following session, he drew a picture which strangely combined things such as a breast, a human brain, and a square sun (**Picture 7**). Under this situation which impressively expressed the objects being fragmented, the patient clearly portrayed a self-image for the first time in the following session. The patient made a clay work in which Stonehenge and a Moai statue were combined. He was satisfied with his performance and wrote mysterious letters on it. Furthermore, he drew a self-image with one leg and protruded lungs (which looked like Stonehenge) (**Picture 8**). He also added his favourite strange-shaped flowers. The patient said that he actually felt he was breathing and said he was satisfied drawing it. I, the therapist interpreted, "It shows that you finally have come to be able to breathe and shows your sensation of being alive, but the boundary of your body is not clear. It expresses that your body is not yet integrated since your internal organs protrude; you cannot stand firmly on your own since your hands and feet are not complete yet; and you still only have one hand for you to hold on to me, the therapist, and your mother."

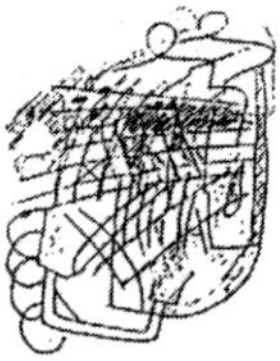

Picture 5

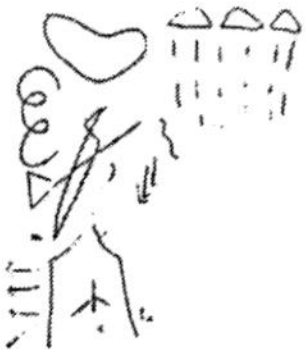

Picture 6

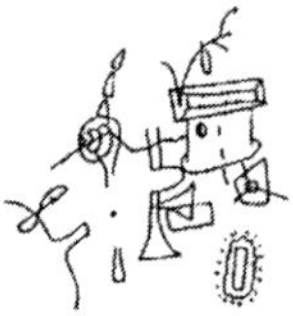

Picture 7

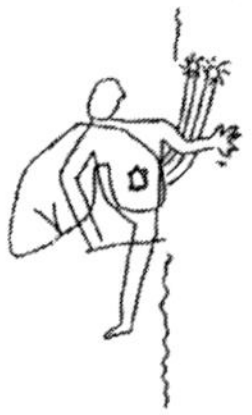

Picture 8

In the following session, the patient drew fragmentary pictures that I did not understand, despite that, he said he had had a dream of having fun playing with children. This is thought to represent that, as Bion said, the patient's ability to dream was gradually recovering and that the non-psychotic part of the mind was starting to activate. The patient then made something which seemed to be two figures with clay and absorbedly played with them over 30 minutes. He stretched the larger figure's arm around the smaller figure's shoulder, variously changed the location of the hands, and connected them at the navel part and abdomens. I interpreted, "This represents not only the relationship between you and your mother, the relationship between the mother and the child, but also the fact that you face me with the feelings of a small child. It also expresses a state where a sexual relationship is also a little mixed up." The patient only gave a little nod as usual.

In the following session, the patient mentioned that he was extremely emotionally dependent on his mother and would smile happily when he saw her face. He then drew a very concrete realistic self-image where he was sitting on an airplane (**Picture 9**). This was a picture that expressed the patient's intention to sit on the airplane, that is treatment, and fly far way together. In addition, the patient used two lumps of clay to express various positional relations. He spent a long time playing the relationships of getting a piggy-back, being cuddled and being breast-fed. Around this time, the therapist observed such world together with the patient, with a surprised feeling about the world the patient expressed.

In the following session, the patient reported a dream again where "he was hand in hand with someone and it seemed that the patient was like a child". Then, he divided the clay into two and made various connections like the last session, and finally connected and fixed the lower abdomens. He said that he wanted to make them connect like a fish and a bird. When the therapist interpreted, "Both of them don't have hands, so they cannot hold hands," the patient nodded. He then drew figures of two people. One was a person who was firmly clinging on a pole, and the other had only one hand and a fish was stuck on its face (**Picture 10**). This was thought to represent two split self-images of the patient. One was a self that had a solid skin boundary and could firmly hold on to things, although it did not have eyes or a nose. The other was a left-behind self-image that could not hold on to anyone like a fish without hands. Birds were also drawn small in the picture.

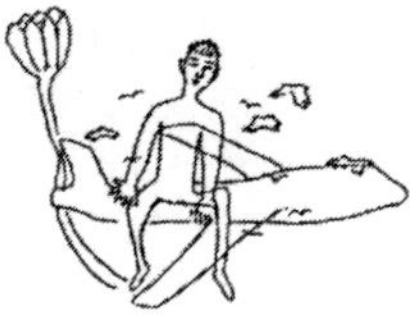

Picture 9

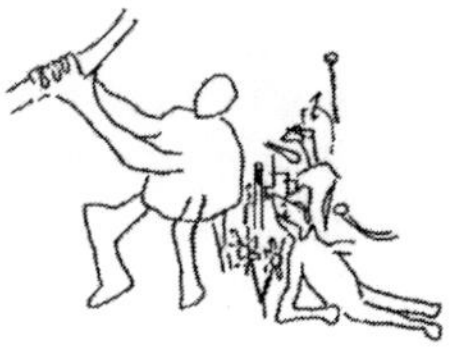

Picture 10

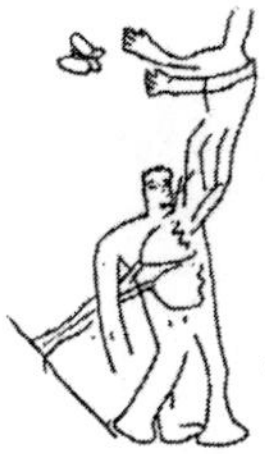

Picture 11

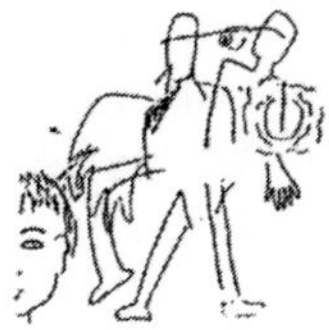

Picture 12

In the following session, the mother who had begun to live with the patient again became angry at the huggy emotional dependence spirit of the patient and went back to her hometown again. At that time, the patient had a dream of "chasing his mother back to her hometown by bicycle". It seemed that although only slightly, a part that could experience object loss existed. Actually, the patient's parents were forcing him to leave university, and he did so later on.

In the following week just before the New Year holidays, the patient said he had a dream in which he was on somebody's shoulders, and also in his picture he drew a person whose hand had become the patient and he was chasing a butterfly (**Picture 11**). This was a picture that indicated well that the patient had fused with the therapist and was about to pursue his goal. Additionally, it could be seen that the patient was trying to reduce his separation anxiety of the New Year holidays, anxiety of leaving university, and anxiety being abandoned by his parents, by fusing with the therapist.

In the first session after the New Year holidays, the patient appeared with an anxious face, and talked that he did not enjoy the New Year holidays very much and that it was decided that he was to drop out of university. He then made a clay figure of a mother bird piggy-backing a baby bird. In addition, he drew a person with two upper bodies, who was receiving energy from the sun, which looked like a female genital organ, and also half of his own face (**Picture 12**). This seems to represent the separation experience with the therapist during the New Year holidays, and the splitting of the patient's self-image and his anxiety concerning the problem of dropping out from university. It expressed that he wanted me, the therapist, to firmly carry him on my back and support him. In the following session, he drew a person going exploring with a new map and expressed his strong will for treatment (**Picture 13**). The world for exploration was a strange space. There was a ladder hanging in mid-air, and things such as an object of a fused male genital organ and female genital organ were soaring. It seemed that exploring inside his mind was equivalent for him to exploring inside the combined body of his parents.

In the following session, the patient said that he went through procedures to leave university. He had a clear face. In clay work, he plunged a knife into a lump of clay and opened a hole saying that it was as if his body was being cut. He then put a small clay ball in it and said "I feel calm now." I interpreted, "This is like a baby entering a tummy. You are feeling that you can feel safe as long as you are like a baby in a mother's body or you are like a baby in the therapist's world, even if you have frictions with your parents regarding your drop out." In the following session, the patient drew a picture where a child firmly holding hands with a person is waving goodbye to another leaving adult (**Picture 14**). This seemed to express the patient's attitude in which he was parting with the world of his university and his parents, and was going to firmly hold on to the therapist.

In addition, around this time, his parents began to recommend the patient to come back to his hometown because of reasons including an economic reason. In the drawing he drew around this time, he drew a big hand and a self-image walking across the boundary (**Picture 15**). Moreover, in clay work, he made something like a big weight. He made a hole in it in the end and said, "I will be troubled if you go far, so I made a hole to keep you tied to it." This was a good expression of the patient's desire to hold on and be tied firmly to the therapist worrying that treatment might end. The patient continued, "I may not be able to come here anymore."

In the following session, the patient reported the following dreams. "There was a traffic accident in a tunnel so I cannot go through. In the other dream, I am right near a pond, but there is no water in the pond. I live with someone on a tree. There was a small house in the middle of the empty pond too and someone lives in it. The pond seemed to be a crater of a volcano." I, the therapist, interpreted that "Your parents collided with me and blocked the way so that you cannot come to treatment." In addition, I interpreted that "When you cannot come for treatment, you go into a state where you dry up. And also, the dream represents that the pond is on a dangerous volcano, that is, treatment is on your parents." Next, he made three arms of a power shovel with clay and connected them. He then said that his father is telling the patient to return to his hometown for economic reasons. The therapist interpreted about the patient being driven by a powerful force such as his father. The patient then drew a mixed picture including a self-image with no arms and feet, a rock musician, and a power shovel (**Picture 16**). I interpreted this that "the patient is in a state where his arms and feet are plucked off by the force of his powerful parents, and the drawing expresses the patient wanting to resist and also himself being driven by a powerful force".

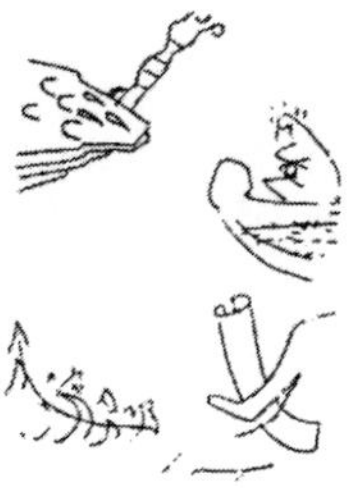
Picture 13

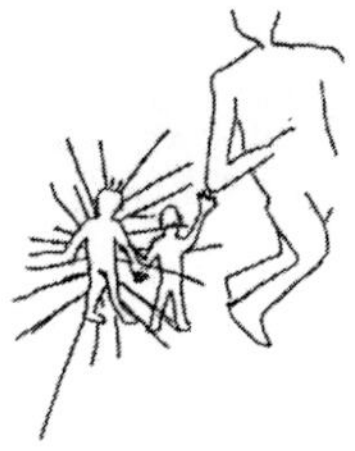
Picture 14

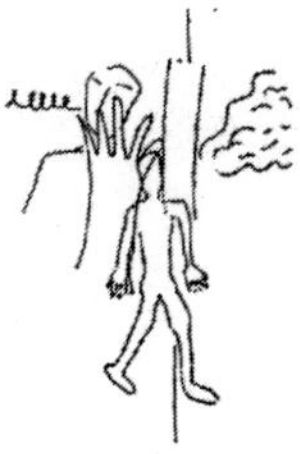
Picture 15

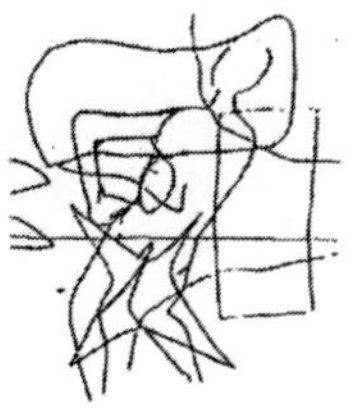
Picture 16

5. Considerations and Conclusion

As described above, the world the patient expressed by drawings and clay works skilfully expressed the fragmented world of his psychotic ego and sometimes the integrated world of his neurotic self. In accordance with the conflicts the patient faced, he sometimes drew pictures and created clay works that brilliantly expressed his body self-image. I, the therapist, maintained an attitude to interpret these as the same method as dream interpretation. There were times when the therapist's interpretations were well understood by the patient, and the patient's drawing expressions and clay expressions developed further on. In such cases, it can be assumed that this expressed that the therapist's approaches were appropriate. When looking at what seems to represent the self-image, when the conflict experienced at that time was psychotic, the object was also fragmented, the body image was not integrated in the self-image, and they mainly indicated an assembly, deficit, and deciduation of body parts, or destruction of the skin boundary. In this way, it can be said that at the psychotic stage of the so-called paranoid-schizoid position, the self-image is not integrated, and is something fragmented. As further integration progressed, it became possible for the patient's drawing to have symbolic expressions and his self-image also became close to being concrete and integrated. He also began to talk about dreams, which represent well the primitive relationship and conflicts with his parents. It seems actually correct to say that the ability to have dreams emerges when the integration of the depressive position has begun to a certain degree. In the actual course, the two positions fluctuate alternately over and over again and move towards a healthy development.

For the method to obtain data on this kind of developmental process of the self body image, materials including drawings of adults in such a psychotic state, and young children's play will be the most important.

References

(1) Bick, Esther. 1968. "The Experience of the Skin in Early Object Relations". *International Journal of Psychoanalysis*, Vol.49: 484-486.

(2) Bion, Wilfred Ruprecht. 1962. *Learning from Experience*. London: Heinemann.

(3) Bion, Wilfred Ruprecht. 1967. *Second Thoughts*. London: Heinemann.

(4) Klein, Melanie. 1932/1975. "Psychoanalysis of children". In *The Writings of Melanie Klein,* Vol.2. London: Hogarth.

(5) Segal, Hanna. 1964. *Introduction to the work of Melanie Klein*. London: Heinemann.

(6) Schilder, Paul. 1935. *The image and appearance of the human body*. London: Kegan & Paul.

[1998. *The Japanese Journal of Psycho-analysis*, Vol. 42, No. 2.]

CHAPTER 4

BORDERLINE PERSONALITY DISORDER: A VIEW OF ENGLISH PSYCHOANALYSIS

1. Introduction

Research on borderline cases have been carried out mainly in the United States. As is well known, studies were conducted on "latent psychosis" from the 1950s, pathological studies on various personality disorders, sexual perversions, addictions in O. Kernberg's [(4)] [(5)] "borderline personality organization" from the late 1960s, and from the early 1980s, studies on "borderline personality disorder" of DSM-III-R and IV, which extract only "emotionally unstable personality disorder", the core patients of "borderline personality organization". In this paper, the term "borderline case" is used as a concept encompassing all studies. In the United Kingdom, when borderline cases are discussed, most of them are about the former two, and "borderline personality disorder" is rarely taken up alone.

In England, the concept of borderline cases was rarely used until Kernberg's studies were introduced. However, clinical researches on various personality disorders, perversions, and addictions, which Kernberg studied under the concept of "borderline personality organization", had already been carried out in the United Kingdom before Kernberg's research and unique pathological theories have been established. They had much influence on Kernberg's studies on borderline cases.

In other words, when describing the studies of borderline cases in the United Kingdom, the American concept cannot be applied as it is, since the studies were conducted under different concepts, and the historical background and patient characteristics of the studies were different. Even if similar patient groups were the target subjects for the clinical researches, the theoretical viewpoints and concepts were different. Therefore, the same term may have different meanings or the target of clinical descriptions may vary so it is a little confusing.

Here, while introducing the history of psychoanalytic clinical research in the United Kingdom, I would like to introduce British researches on so-called "borderline cases", and their influence on Kernberg's research of "borderline personality organization" and the British analysts' criticisms on it. By doing so, the position of the study on "borderline cases" in the United Kingdom will be clarified.

2. Research on borderline psychosis

The first to use this concept was J. Rickman and analysts such as W. Bion [(2)] adopted it, too. Patients with borderline psychosis refers to a group of patients who develop a psychotic breakdown during the course of psychoanalytic treatment while receiving medical consultation for neurotic symptoms. Borderline psychosis generally corresponds to the concept of latent psychosis represented by R. Knight's study. Studies on psychoanalysis for manic-depressive illness had already started in the United Kingdom in the 1930s, and pathologically severe patients had been treated from a very early stage. In addition, from the 1940s, M. Klein and her disciples including Bion, H. Rosenfeld and H. Segal began therapeutic research on psychoanalysis for schizophrenia and, as part of it, conducted clinical research on patients with borderline psychosis. In that sense, borderline psychosis had been actively selected as a therapeutic target for psychoanalysis as part of the studies on schizophrenia.

Then, in the 1950s, analysts gradually began to deal with patients with severe personality disorders such as sexual perversion, addiction, schizoid, narcissism, and impulsive disorder. In that sense, in the United Kingdom, studies on so-called borderline cases moved from clinical studies on severe psychosis to studies in mild patient groups.

The characteristics of the internal object relations in the concept of Kernberg's research on "borderline personality organization" take on those of Klein's schizoid mechanism. Therefore, when Kernberg's study on borderline cases was published in 1967, it was accepted in the United Kingdom without any sense of incongruity.

3. Klein's psychoanalysis for children (1920-1932 [(6)])

Klein, especially under the auspices of K. Abraham conducted psychoanalysis for young children aged 2-3 years, who were not considered to be targets for psychoanalysis at the time. She found that the play of such young children also had the function of communication to express themselves just like free association of adults. Klein discovered that the world expressed there indicated that the inner world of such young children already existed, and called the unconscious world as "unconscious phantasy". This world represents the disposition of infancy (0-year-olds), and part object relations and primitive defence mechanisms, including splitting, projection, introjection, denial, idealization, and omnipotence, are active there. In that world, the oral phase sadism and anal phase sadism are dominant, and it is a world dominated by strong love and persecutory anxiety. In other words, infants regard the object which gives them satisfaction (the mother) as a "good object" and idealize it and direct strong love towards it. On the contrary, infants regard the object that gives them frustration (the mother) as a "bad object". The infants violently attack the bad object and conversely suffer from persecutory anxiety fearing that they may be retaliated. They are not yet able to recognize that these contradictory part-objects are different sides of the same object, due to the mechanism of splitting. Klein proposed that this world of primitive object relations was transferred in psychoanalytic treatment, and by verbally interpreting the anxiety, the analyst can bring about changes to the patient. The world of early unconscious phantasies discovered through this became a basic perspective for the later studies on adult psychosis and personality disorders. Subsequently, it had a great influence on Kernberg's concept of "borderline personality organization".

4. Klein's study on manic depressive illness and the "depressive position" (1935-1945 [7] [8])

In the 1930s, Klein conducted psychoanalytic studies on adult manic-depressive illness. This was a continuation of Abraham's study [1]. S. Freud believed that manic-depressive illness, schizophrenia, and paranoia were not subject to psychoanalysis because they were narcissistic neuroses that did not develop transferences.

Klein took in much of Abraham's opinion and considered that the pathological fixation point of manic-depressive illness was in the conflict world of object relations from the late oral stage to the early anal stage. She called this the "depressive position". This is related to the timing of transition from part object relation to whole object relation. Its origin is in the object relation of infants from about 6 months old. Around that time, babies gradually come to know that what were part objects until then due to the mechanism of splitting, the "good object" and the "bad object", are actually two sides of the same mother. At that time, infants become aware that the good object, which they strongly loved, and the bad object, which they had directed intense hatred to and which had made them shiver with persecuted anxiety, were the same object. Infants then experience a strong conflict as they realize they had been violently attacking their beloved object. The conflict includes the fear of losing their object and the feeling of guilt for attacking the object. This is the infants' world of experiencing "object loss". The defence mechanisms working here are mitigated ones where splitting, projection, introjection, and denial can be seen. Manic defence is seen, too. J. Steiner, who will be described later, considers that in the depressive state often seen in borderline cases, the patients transiently have the above experiences.

5. Fairbairn's study on the schizoid mechanism (1940s-early 1950s [(3)])

D. Fairbairn was inspired by Abraham's developmental theory and Klein's "paranoid position" (Klein later came to call it as the "paranoid schizoid position") and "depressive position" (1935), and developed his own personality theory and pathology. He first focused on hysteria, suggesting that the issue of splitting of the ego and the object in the early oral stage played a major role. He came to find that it had a great deal to do with schizoid personality, manic-depressive illness, and schizophrenia. Furthermore, he advocated that neurosis was a technique used when patients were unable to cope with psychotic anxiety and depressive anxiety associated with those splittings, and that there were four methods: hysteria, compulsion, phobia, and paranoia. In contrast to Klein et al. who studied the schizoid mechanic from the studies on psychosis, Fairbairn studied neurosis and advanced to studying the schizoid mechanism.

The developmental personality theory based on his schizoid mechanism is as follows. New born babies are object-seeking from the beginning, and repeatedly experience satisfaction and frustration at first mainly through suckling. Babies introject the frustrating bad object, repress it with the associated ego, and place it in their unconsciousness. This bad object is called an "exciting object" in the sense that it stimulates, excites, but does not satisfy the baby. The corresponding part of the ego becomes satisfied by such suckling of the breast but at the same time, becomes anxious that he/she might destroy the object. Fairbairn called such an ego as the "libidinal ego". This corresponds to the suckling period in the early oral period. However, by the time the babies' teeth begin to grow in the latter half of 0-year-olds, the frustrating object is experienced as something to reject, and the babies respond to such object with destructive attacks of biting and ripping, and begin to suffer from depressive anxiety that they have lost the object. Fairbairn named such an object as a "rejecting object" and the corresponding ego as the "internal saboteur" (later "antilibidinal ego"). In this way, Fairbairn considered that object relations in infancy influenced the basis of their personality formation. He said that infants dealt with the relation with their first bad object by introjecting it, splitting it, and foreclosing it into their unconsciousness, and that such bad objects come in the above-mentioned two types; an exciting object and a rejecting object.

On the contrary, according to Fairbairn, infants do not introject the object that gives good satisfaction at first but idealizes it and then makes the ego which is experiencing the corresponding satisfaction their central ego.

Thus, Fairbairn advocated that what becomes the core of personality depends on extremely early object relations. If the bad object relation is too strong at this stage, the associated delusional anxiety and depressive anxiety also become stronger and have various adverse influences on personality development. If the problem with the "exciting object" is too strong, predisposition for future schizophrenia remains, and if the ambivalent conflict with the "rejecting object" is too strong, the predisposition for manic-depressive illness will remain. When those anxieties are not extreme, the above neurotic techniques are skilfully used and they clinically appear as neurosis.

Fairbairn called the above mechanism as the schizoid mechanism, and was interested in the "schizoid personality", which was thought to be a clinical manifestation of the relationship with such objects. Patients with schizoid personality deal with internal anxieties and conflicts by disconnecting their relationships with others. Their characteristics include withdrawal, interest in their self, and facts centred on ideas in their own world. He also states that this schizoid state is found in other cases which show diverse clinical manifestations. It is considered that Kernberg's borderline patients are included in this.

Actually, there is something in common between Fairbairn's idea, that there is a schizoid mechanism behind the many symptoms of clinical diseases and that it is important to therapeutically handle that part of the split bad object relation, and Kernberg's idea of "borderline personality organization". Kernberg himself stated that he was influenced by works by not only M. Maler, E. Jacobson, and Klein but also Fairbairn's works while he was studying borderline cases.

It is also noteworthy that representative researchers of borderline cases, such as J. Masterson and D. Rinsley, have taken in Fairbairn's schizoid studies.

6. Klein's study on schizophrenia and the "paranoid-schizoid position" (1946) [9]

From the 1940s, Klein began conducting analytical studies on schizophrenia and published them in 1946 as studies on the "schizoid mechanism". Klein found there again that early object relation, which was discovered in children's psychoanalysis, was involved in the mechanism. This means that the fixation point of schizophrenia is related to the disposition of 3 to 4-month-old babies. It is a part object relation, and primitive defence mechanisms of splitting, projection, introjection, denial, idealization, and additionally, projective identification are active. Babies split the good and the bad objects so they cannot recognize that they are the same object. Then, the babies idealize the good object and directs strong love towards it. On the other hand, they direct violent attacks and hatred towards the bad object, and become terrified by the anxiety of being retaliated, that is, persecutory anxiety. Klein called this the "paranoid-schizoid position". (When Klein proposed the concept of the "depressive position" in 1935, she predicted an earlier stage and called it the "paranoid position" but she came to call it the "paranoid-schizoid position" taking in Fairbairn's opinion.) Klein considered that the unprocessed and split-off remains in the unconsciousness of the state where the bad object relation overwhelms have great relevancy to schizophrenia. These are also Klein's study on the schizoid mechanism. Klein's studies were taken over without any modification as a description of the inner world, represented by Kernberg's splitting in "borderline personality organization", and has had a great influence on current studies on borderline cases. More importantly, such Klein's studies resulted from the studies on schizophrenia, and later it was revealed that there exists a similar mechanism in pathologically mild personality disorders.

7. Development of clinical research on schizophrenia

From the mid-1940s to the 1960s, studies on schizophrenia were further developed by Bion, Rosenfeld, Segal [14] and other analysts. In particular, Bion conducted studies on psychotic personality, thought, projective identification, and container/contained. Furthermore, as shown above, analysts conducted research on psychoanalytic treatment for latent psychosis based on the concept of borderline psychosis.

8. Winnicott's study on "false self" (19)

D. Winnicott hardly used the term "borderline cases", and did not write much about patients with emotionally unstable personality disorder, who fall into the core group of borderline patients. However, he conducted studies on "false self", which is similar to the "as-if personality", which is considered to be a subtype of borderline cases. False-self is a part of the so-called over-adapted self. The patients with false-self superficially seem to be adapted to society, but actually have many unresolved conflicts in the background. They cannot face their original conflicting problems unless this excessive "false self" defensive action is processed. Winnicott, like other British analysts, believed that the conflict originated in infancy holding (from birth up to 6 months of age) and the period of concerns (6 months to 2 years of age).

9. Rosenfeld's study on "destructive narcissistic organization" (1960-1970s) (12) (13)

From the 1960s, Kleinian studies on schizophrenia eclipsed a little. Kleinians began to study various personality disorders such as sexual perversion, addiction, schizoid, as-if, and impulsive personality, and began to pay attention to the specific "defence organization" (Segal, E. O'Shaughnessy (10)). This developed to the following studies of Rosenfeld and Steiner, and then to the borderline theory in the United Kingdom. The patient groups in these studies are almost the same as the patient groups studied in Kernberg's "borderline personality organization".

Rosenfeld moved from studying schizophrenia to studying patients with various personality disorders, perversions, and addictions. He considered that there was a unique defence organization in the inner world of such patients, and called it a "destructive narcissistic organization". This is a study on the primitive superego in the inner world of such patients, and a study on a defence organization. Such patients are patients who show a so-called negative treatment reaction where the treatment itself is stagnated or interrupted, and when the treatment is about to succeed, the patients show destructive acting-out such as suicide, crime, or self-mutilation.

According to Rosenfeld, in such patients, the self introjects a destructive object into a part of the mind, and a part is formed which violently controls the other parts of self, like a Mafia. It attacks and destroys other dependent parts of the self which seek the object. Moreover, such a destructive part is idealized and identifies with the self. Excitement and perversion occur there, and the self idealizes the destructing of the object. By doing so, the self prevents the good relationship with the object to evolve and impedes the mind to develop. Rosenfeld considered that envy played a major role in the formation of such an organization. This was a development of Klein's study on envy and negative therapeutic responses, and a development of the study on primitive superego.

In 1978, Rosenfeld took up and criticized Kernberg's "borderline personality organization", which had become known worldwide. This was the first time this concept was actively taken up in the United Kingdom. Rosenfeld gave a consideration on the pathology of "borderline personality organization" from the perspective of "destructive narcissistic organization", which has become one of the representatives of British borderline theories.

L. Sohn also studied the problem of pathological narcissism from the perspective of the pathology of "introjection", and has caused a stir in the study of borderline cases.

10. Rey's commentary on "borderline personality organization" (1979) (11) (16)

H. Rey understood the concept of "borderline personality organization" as Klein's "schizoid mechanism", and considered that it was seen not only in the patient groups advocated by Kernberg, but also in patients who corrupt as schizophrenia or manic-depressive illness, patients with hysterical personalities, and patients with obsessive-compulsive personalities. He took up case patients who fell into a transient psychotic condition, and proposed that this was developmentally related to the disposition of a 0-year-old baby. Rey criticized Kernberg's perspective on Mahler's theory and reviewed the "borderline personality organization" through the original Klein's "paranoid-schizoid position" theory.

11. Steiner's concept of "pathological organization" (1980s) (16)-(18)

Steiner conducted studies on the robust defence organization commonly found in personality disorders such as schizoid personality, psychotic personality, borderline personality, sexual perversion, and addiction. Steiner was particularly influenced by Rosenfeld's work. He called the defence organization as "pathological organization", and proposed that it was a pathological defence organization that partially had properties of object relation and primitive defence mechanism which are seen in the "paranoid-schizoid position" and "depressive position". Pathological organization is created when envy and aggression are projectively identified with the object, and the fragments of them are re-introjected into the self, and fused. It is a world of addictive and perverted object relations, which struggles to flatly resist change, tries to maintain equilibrium, and works as a complex defence organization. It has a great impact on the pathological aspect of personality. Seemingly, since it is similar to the "paranoid-schizoid position" or the "depressive position", it is mistaken for them. However, in fact, it works as a strong defence against the two positions, and is a defence against healthy persecutory anxiety and depressive anxiety. It also interferes with the process of object loss and prevents mental development. This organization can also be called the third position, and it exists at the borderline between the "paranoid-schizoid position" and the "depressive position". In this way, Steiner clarified what was once not clear: the distinction between the normal position and the pathological position. He considered that the property of this "pathological organization" was highly diverse, some are extremely severely psychotic and some are neurotic, such as obsessive-compulsive. Although Steiner conceived that pathological organization was seen in a wider range of illnesses than in Kernberg's Borderline cases, from psychosis to neurosis, the pathological organization is an organization where the aspect as a defence organization is emphasized. Steiner stated that both of Kernberg's "borderline personality organization" and "borderline personality disorder" were a type of this "pathological organization".

12. Conclusion

As seen above, while introducing the history of British psychoanalysis in chronological order, I described the influence of it on Kernberg's study of borderline cases, that is, "borderline personality organization", and the impact on the establishment of "borderline personality disorder" in DSM-III-R, IV.

In the United Kingdom, research on manic-depressive illness and schizophrenia had been conducted since the 1930s, and the theory of early development of "depressive position" and "paranoid-schizoid position" was established. This theory of primitive object relations, which is based on splitting and projective identification, had a great influence on Kernberg's theory of "borderline personality organization".

From the 1940s, there was Fairbairn's research on the schizoid mechanism, which had a great influence not only on Kernberg but also on American borderline researchers such as Masterson.

In the United Kingdom, analytical studies on various personality disorders, perversion, and addiction began to be conducted from the 1960s onward, and unique pathologies developed. These include Winnicott's "false self," Rosenfeld's "destructive narcissistic organization," and Steiner's "pathological organization". Although they include a slightly wider patient population than the patient population associated to Kernberg's "borderline personality organization", the studies were conducted in almost a common patient population. It can be said that they are unique pathologies of British borderline studies.

References

(1) Abraham, Karl. 1927. *Selected Papers of Karl Abraham, M. D.* London: Hogarth Press and Institute of Psychoanalysis.

(2) Bion, Wilfred. 1967. *Second Thoughts*. London: Heinemann.

(3) Fairbairn, W. Ronald. D. 1952. *Psychoanalytic Studies of the Personality*. London: Routledge.

(4) Kernberg, Otto. 1967. "Borderline Personality Organization". *Journal of American Psychoanalytic Association*, 15: 641-685.

(5) Kernberg, Otto. 1975. *Borderline Conditions and Pathological Narcissism*. New York: Jason Aronson.

(6) Klein, Melanie. 1932/1975. "Psychoanalysis of Children". In *The Writings of Melanie Klein*, Vol. 2. London: Hogarth Press.

(7) Klein, Melanie. 1935/1975. "A Contribution to the Psychogenesis of Manic-Depressive States". In *The Writings of Melanie Klein*, Vol. 1. London: Hogarth Press.

(8) Klein, Melanie. 1490/1975. "Mourning and Its Relation to Manic-Depressive States". In *The Writings of Melanie Klein*, Vol. 1, 344-369. London: Hogarth Press.

(9) Klein, Melanie. 1946/1975. "Notes on Some Schizoid Mechanisms". In *The Writings of Melanie Klein*, Vol. 3, 1-24. London: Hogarth Press.

(10) O'Shaughnessy, Edna. 1981. "A Clinical Study of a Defensive Organization". *International Journal of Psychoanalysis*, 62: 359-369.

(11) Rey, Henri. 1979/1988. "Schizoid Phenomena in the Borderline". In *Melanie Klein Today*, Vol. 1, edited by Elizabeth Bott Spillius. London: Routledge.

(12) Rosenfeld, Herbert. 1964/1965. "On the Psychopathology of Narcissism: A Clinical approach". In *Psychotic States*. London: Hogarth Press.

(13) Rosenfeld, Herbert. 1971. "A Clinical Approach to the Psychoanalytic Theory of the Life and Death Instincts: An Investigation into the

Aggressive Aspects of Narcissism". *International Journal of Psychoanalysis*, 52: 169-178.
(14) Segal, Hanna. 1981. *The Work of Hanna Segal*. London: Jason Aronson.
(15) Sohn, Leslie. 1985/1988. "Narcissistic Organization, Projective Identification and the Formation of the Identificate". *Melanie Klein Today*, Vol. l, edited by Elizabeth Bott Spillius. London: Routledge.
(16) Edited. by Spillius, Elizabeth Bott. 1988. *Melanie Klein Today*, Vol. l. London: Routledge.
(17) Steiner, John. 1979. "The Border Between the Paranoid-Schizoid and the Depressive Positions in the Borderline Patients". *British Journal of Medical Psychology*, 52 (4): 385-391.
(18) Steiner, John. 1993. *Psychic Retreats*. London: Routledge.
(19) Winnicott, Donald Woods. 1965. "The Maturational Processes and the Facilitating Environment". *International Psycho-Analytical Library*, 64: 1-278.

[1996. *Review of Psychiatry*, Vol. 20.]

CHAPTER 5

A CASE PATIENT WITH A FLASHBACK OF SEXUALLY TRAUMATIZED EXPERIENCE IN HER CHILDHOOD

1. Introduction

In recent years, American researchers have been studying cases with post-traumatic stress disorder. Among them, cases with the problem of sexual abuse in early childhood are also considered. I, the author would like to report my experience treating a patient who had suffered symptoms including depressive anxiety attacks since she had a sudden flashback at the age of 19 about a childhood rape incident. Since this is mainly a case report, I would like to focus on the therapeutic process and techniques, and minimize literature consideration.

2. Case

Patient T was a 22-year-old woman at the initial visit and was a second-generation Japanese of Country A (Her main language was English). When she was 19, she was listening to her friend talk about sexual abuse, and she suddenly recalled a memory of being raped by an unknown man when she was five, and she began to suffer from a depressive state, anxiety attacks, and a feeling of victimhood. She went to a psychiatric clinic and she started taking antidepressants and anxiolytics and had continued to take them until she came to see me, the therapist, for the initial visit. At the age of 20, a heartbreak triggered her to develop minor wrist-cutting behaviour. She said she had little memory of her childhood, but she faintly remembered being spanked often by her father and being bullied by her sister. T said that she knew for the first time that her mother had schizophrenia when she became a high school student, and that the mystery of her mother's strange behaviour was solved. T had one older brother and one older sister. In Country A, she participated in a rape victim group but discontinued it, and instead received instructional counselling once every two weeks. However, she felt there was no change. She then came to Japan alone, hoping to find a new direction. She decided to go to a language school while staying at her aunt's house and helping her work. However, even after she came to Japan, her symptoms such as depression, anxiety attacks, and interpersonal tension worsened, thus she was referred to me. The exacerbation of these symptoms was thought to be related to the reaction for the loss of leaving her home country.

(1) Introduction period: 1st to 9th session

After four diagnostic interviews, she began to receive psychoanalytic psychotherapy once-a-week with a face-to-face method.

At first, patient T told the therapist that she was mistaken for a bicycle thief by a police officer, and that people would not readily believe what she said. She also said that she was misleading and was isolated because she had a distance with others, and that what she said might have a negative effect on others. The therapist interpreted that leaving her home country and coming to an unfamiliar country must have been extremely lonesome, and that what she told the therapist represented well that, upon starting treatment, she was worried if the therapist would understand and believe her, and that she might be influenced badly by the therapist. In response, T expressed her concern that she could not believe anyone and that neither other people nor the therapist would believe in her. This in itself represented T's typical early transference when encountering a stranger therapist during the introduction period. In addition, T also expressed her anxiety that if she started talking about herself, she might start crying and might not be able to stop. T also said, "I do not want to think about my life and if I did, it would make people feel uncomfortable." Here, it seemed that T had foreseen that she would come to speak of her own conflicting world of life if she received therapy.

However, on the other hand, T said, "My father did not try to save me at all, and my mother was always taken care of by me." She continued, "My sister ran away quickly, and no one saved me. I have lived feeling that I was a very bad child if I couldn't solve the problems of my mother and my family." This story expressed T's transference feelings that even if she talked about herself to the therapist, the therapist would not even try to rescue her nor take responsibility. Around this time, T often smiled while she told such stories. When the therapist pointed it out, T began to talk crying bitterly. In addition, the therapist mentioned how hard a life T had lived feeling that it was her responsibility although what she had tried to do was an extremely impossible and heavy burden for a little child.

In the next session, T told that her depression was exacerbating and she had suicidal ideation. She then said she had started writing letters to her family and was writing a lot of complaints. She also told the therapist that her family would just make demands to her and no one had helped her. In this way, T felt that by starting receiving therapy, she had no other choice but to talk about her painful experience about her family. However, talking her experiences struck her with a terrible feeling of despair and suicidal ideation. She would often smile then, too, and when the therapist pointed that out, T sobbed bitterly and complained about her family. After she told those complaints, she said, "I become filled with loathing because I become empty and feel that it's meaningless." She then said with claims against the therapist, "People cannot change my reality."

Thereafter, although she suffered, she began to recall her past. According to her memory, in the past, her father strangled her and she fainted and lost her subsequent memory. She asked herself, "What the hell happened?" Furthermore, her father tried to make T work even the day after the day T attempted suicide when she was 20 years old. T said that her father just made demands to her and did not do anything for her. She also expressed her anxiety that she might be thought she was crazy if she said things like that. In addition, T recalled that, from her childhood, her father called her mother a mad person, and he often said that T was also like her mother. T said, "Telling you such things doesn't give me any hope or help. It is meaningless and only increases hopelessness." The therapist stated that T was worried that people would think that she was a mad person even if she just had or spoke her natural feelings, and that she was not able to sort her feelings out because she was overwhelmed. The therapist also interpreted that T felt that the therapist had an aspect which did not try to save her, just like her parents. Around this time, T showed injurious behaviour where she would lightly cut her body with a razor.

T insisted that she could not control her madness and that there was no solution, and said she wanted to know more about Buddhism. The therapist told T that she was telling her disappointment and criticism against treatment and interpreted that she was looking for something like Buddhism that would provide her an omnipotent remedy. The therapist advised her to continue this treatment. Continuously, T talked about her family and said that her father did not believe her even after she was raped. T also said that her sister did not save her, rather she touched T's body and hurt her. T then cried intensely that no one would help her. She began to complain that she got strange looks from people and said that she was staying still locked up in her room because people were treacherous. The therapist considered that this expressed T's defensive attitude: T foreclosed herself, who would ask for help when she was really in trouble, and tried to solve the problems by withdrawing in suspicion and disappointment to avoid the problems. Thus, the therapist interpreted as so.

(2) 2nd period: The period when T showed even stronger anxiety about touching her inner world; 10th to 18th session

T began to appeal that she wanted to become a nun and help others. She also said, "People cannot understand me. They abuse and reject me." The therapist interpreted that T actually wanted the therapist and others to take care of her and save her like a nun. T sobbed and recalled with confused and intense emotions that when she was being raped, she was pushed down on a mat and although she called her father, he did not reply. She then talked about her hopeless feelings that no one saved her, saying "I want to leave the therapy room. I have nothing more to say." The therapist told T that she felt that no one, not even the therapist, could do anything when she was in so much trouble, and that she felt people were pretending not to be able to hear when she asked for help. T told the therapist, "You can do nothing more. I feel desperate and have no hope." The therapist clarified that such feelings had begun to become more apparent those days, and she was experiencing pain as she recalled various things. Furthermore, the therapist interpreted that T had long sought a person who would listen to and understand her painful feelings, but when she got an opportunity to receive treatment in reality, she felt stronger frustration, could not feel its valuable aspect and could not take advantage of the opportunity.

In the following session, T said, "I want to change the treatment frequency to once every two weeks. Treatment is not helpful and I have nothing to talk about." She continued, "I already told my friend about myself, but it didn't help. I want to move to an apartment and live alone." In addition, T said, "I have tried to removed what actually happened in reality considering it as a dream or paralyzing my senses," and said she wanted to be a nun, again. The therapist intervened that T thought that no realistic person could save her, and wanted a dedicated person like a nun to help her. The therapist also said that T was so dissatisfied that she did not want to admit that she was actually getting help at the treatment site.

Furthermore, in the following session, T said, "I want to reduce treatment to once a month. I want to live alone in an apartment." The therapist reiterated interpretations such that when T asked someone for help, she always felt dissatisfied like that and would eventually leave the person and withdraw into herself, and that she knew that method did not work. The therapist also thought that T saw in the therapist an aspect of her father who ignored and refused to save her, and she was attacking and refusing that part. The therapist told her that she should come every week. Then, T made a remark which symbolically appreciated the supportive part of the therapist, "At least the medicine you, the therapist, prescribed is effective and alleviates my anxiety."

Thereafter, T's sister sent a letter to T saying that she wanted to live with T. That made T happy. She stopped moving out to an apartment and said she wanted to continue to live with her aunt. This was related to the fact that T was glad of the therapist's intervention and she had a feeling to accept them.

T was smiling at the time, but she began to look at the world of her self again and recalled the rape incident. She said that her father would just keep saying bad things about her, and he ignored her when she was raped, too. She also told the therapist that the doctor who examined T at that time was kind enough to report it to the police. Symbolic signs that T was beginning to trust the therapist could be seen again in her words, but on the other hand, it seemed that she was also projecting a negative-example-father-like terrible human image. T said, "When I attempted suicide two years ago, I was triggered by a heartbreak from a man who looked a lot like the man who raped me." However, she complained, "My father didn't understand my suffering."

The start time of the following session was changed. T got the times mixed up and appeared at the wrong time, and the therapist was not there. In the following session, she appealed her loneliness and told the therapist that she had kept on crying alone at home. She said her sense of loneliness was strong, and it was first time since she attempted suicide two years ago that she felt so. She then complained, "I don't want to rely on other people. Other people are cold. I don't want to say anything. I can't believe in people. My father didn't care about me, either." The therapist gave a transference interpretation that T felt that way against the therapist because he changed the time and took an attitude of ignoring her.

(3) 3rd period: Period when T gradually started to accept help from the therapist and her sister; 19th to 25th session

Thereafter, T continued saying, "My sister wrote me a letter saying that she wanted to live with me, but I can't believe if she really thinks so." The therapist interpreted that even though T knew that other people were really thinking about her, she did not want to admit it because she was angry. She complained, "Why did my sister touch my body and hurt me back then?" She then told the therapist that her sister had written the following dream in her letter: "My sister pushed T out of a window. My sister hung from a tree in front of their parents' room and was stabbing herself with something sharp." T said, "I wrote to my sister that the dream represented her guilt towards me," and told the therapist, "I can't believe that my family is worried about me." The therapist intervened, "Even if you realize that you are receiving help from people, it seems that you do not want to admit that. That is probably because you are angry and have a sense of hopelessness."

In the next session, T mentioned that her life had become a little more enjoyable, that Japanese was difficult and she wanted to study it more, and that she also wanted to learn Buddhism. At the same time, T began to think about returning to her country and began to confirm with her sister if she really wanted to live with T. She also felt the kindness of her aunt and came to be able to accept it. This episode represent that T had accepted the therapist's value and that she was trying to accept the experiences in the treatment. She also said that when she received a phone call from her father, she was able to speak in Japanese for the first time and felt him closer, but she could not forgive him. From this time on, T came to be able to feel her feelings distinctly and her facial expression became clearer. She then began to clearly and strongly feel her anger towards her family, and at the same time began to feel that she had become quite calm. The therapist gave an interpretation that T had begun to feel her original natural feelings and anger and that actually she had felt them since she was a child but had denied them because she was overwhelmed by and could not cope with them. T said, "I have calmed down at work and at home, but now I am so angry about being abused, being made to work by my father, and being made to take care of my mother. I also cannot help feeling angry about my brother and others just doing what they wanted." In addition, she began to make statements that she had come to indirectly evaluate what the therapist had given her, saying that she should have taken part in the previous rape victim group.

(4) Termination period: Period where symptoms relapsed, defence mechanisms reactivated and self-understanding deepened in the relationship with the therapist; 26th to 36th session

However, from the following session, the time was changed to an evening time due to T's request. T felt that the therapist was tired and did not answer properly, and she developed depression, despair, and a desire to withdraw again. She recalled that her mad mother would violently attack her, would suddenly go missing, and would cause a great deal of trouble to her, and said she could not believe in anyone. Here, it seems that the unstable mother image was transferred to the therapist as he would suddenly lose concentration sometimes. T's such sensitive transference reactions changed drastically during the sessions. She began to say in tears that when she thought about the fact that her father abused her mother, the fact that she needed to help her mother, and her anxieties about the future, she would after all have to deal with them by herself. In addition, when the therapist was late for a session for some reason, T vividly portrayed the experience of being abandoned by the therapist, recalling that her father left her behind in an unfamiliar town because she said something selfish. T agreed when the therapist interpreted it in relation to the nearest time change, and said, "I cannot trust you anymore, too." The therapist interpreted that T's words expressed that her expectations for the therapist were actually becoming even higher, and that she did not want to admit that she was receiving help because she was angry. T continued to complain, "None of my friends, groups members, you, no one understands me." The therapist gave a defence interpretation that when T was angry, she did not want to admit what she was gaining from others, and she wanted to break the relationships and shut herself up. She replied, “I realize that I am always angry lately and when I am alone, I recall various scenes where I was angry when I was a child." Around that time, the therapist got the impression that T's facial expressions were clearer and the emotions she was experiencing were distinct. T began to say again that she had a hard time being made to work by her father and taking care of her mother, but she said she could clearly feel how she felt and how she was angry at the time. She came to say, "I feel I am much better these days and have come to be able to do without medication."

Thereafter, she told the therapist that she felt relieved when she told everything to a foreign friend she had met recently, but when she was asked out to go shopping, she suddenly wanted to keep a distance and withdraw. Furthermore, when the therapist cancelled a session, she said in the following session, "I recalled the terrible things my father did to me one after another in a daydream and I am trying to forget them." When the therapist said it had something to do with the therapist doing a terrible thing by cancelling a session, T agreed and said, "I have begun to have a strong distrust against the therapist." She continued saying that she was staying at home, not wanting to see anyone. The therapist interpreted that that was the main coping method T had been doing for a long time, and that at such times, this therapy and the help and care she received from others would disappear somewhere.

T seemed to have understood the interpretation well. In the following week, she said she was in good shape and thought she could manage to do things alone. She began to associate with her friends again and was able to join in a group at language school and talk about herself. She said, "I don't think I'll shut myself up anymore. I would like to try without receiving treatment for about a month and if it works, I want to go on without treatment." The subsequent course was good, and she suddenly began to wear makeup. She appeared in an adult-like appearance and thanked the therapist. The course after that was good and she finished treatment.

3. Consideration

In his review on post-traumatic stress disorder, Okano described that the disorder of patients like the one in this paper is also a form of post-traumatic disorder, that is, the disorder of patients who develop neurotic symptoms such as strong depression and anxiety attacks because they were sexually traumatized in their childhood and recall their abusive experience in flashbacks when they become adolescents.

I was especially interested in the meaning the traumatic memory, which flashed back as childhood memories, had on T's pathological conflict and onset. First, there is one question: Was the memory true? As far as I listened to this patient, it seems that she actually had such an experience, but rather than questioning whether the memory was true or not, it was much more important for T's treatment to grasp it as a psychic reality.

In other words, the memory functions like a kind of screen memory, and it can be considered that such memory symbolically represented T's conflicting experience from her childhood. It seems there is something in common with the function of dreams. T may have constituted her memory by using the same mechanisms as found in the dream mechanism, such as condensation, displacement, and symbolism of the world of T's inner conflict. T's world of internal conflict was generally made up of painful experiences where she was hurt and attacked by her parents and others.

With this flashback, T's over-adaptive "false self" defence collapsed and she developed depression, anxiety attacks, and a sense of being stared at. In addition, her depression worsened and she attempted suicide after being in an unrequited love with and rejected by a man who looked a lot like the person who T believed to have raped her. This is considered to be a self-deprecating repetitive compulsion for the traumatic experience.

Looking at the actual course of treatment, T began to recall many childhood conflicts with her parents, and the traumatic experience which came back to her mind through flashbacks was only a part of them. The content of T's conflicts was consisted of the facts that she was responsible for taking care of her alcohol-dependent violent father and her unreliable mentally-ill mother, and feelings of desperate depression and hatred against people including her parents who would hurt each other and her siblings. Furthermore, she talked about memories that made the therapist think that it was her father who raped her, but in any case, it was impossible to pursue whether it was true or not, and therapeutically it was more important to understand the dynamics of the psychic fact. The therapist had a strong impression that the flashbacks led T to treatment, reminded her of the various unresolved conflicts with her parents, and provided her an opportunity to resolve them. In other words, flashbacks acted like an entrance to turn her eyes towards her conflicting inner world.

T had dealt with them by suppressing them, erasing them from her memory, excluding emotions and paralyzing her feelings. Additionally, because of the despair against no one helping her and the disappointment and anger against others, T became depressed and suicidal when she began to recall her family problems. On the other hand, she refused help from the therapist, thought it was worthless, and tried to live by herself. This was a typical transference caused by projective identification of T's bad object, and was a defence mechanism of hikikomori. In actual treatment, the most important therapeutical technique was to carefully give transference interpretations on T's distrustful object and interpret T's typical defence mechanism. This is basically the same as the techniques for other neurotic treatment.

Despite showing strong emotional confusion and robust defence, T improved in a relatively short period of time. This is because 1) T's social function had relatively developed despite the aspect of over-adaptation, and she had continued to study while taking care of her parents until the flashback occurred; 2) the way of onset was acute and responsive; 3) it could be considered that a part of her unconsciousness protruded into her world of consciousness due to flashbacks at around the same timing when she began trying to look at her previously unresolved suppressed world; and 4) on the whole, she was probably at a level of mild emotionally unstable personality disorder.

4. Conclusion

I reported the course of treatment of a woman who was considered to have experienced sexual trauma at an early age and who developed depression, anxiety attacks, sense of being stared at, and suicidal ideation triggered by flashbacks during adolescence. I also showed that the treatment is basically the same as the treatment for general neurosis and personality disorders.

References

1) Maruta, Toshihiko. 1995. "Psychic Trauma and Psychic Reality". *Japanese Journal of Psychiatric Treatment,* Vol. 10, No. 1: 3-8 (in Japanese)
2) Okano, Kenichiro. 1995a. *Traumatic Mental Disorders*. Tokyo: Iwasaki Academic Publisher (in Japanese)
3) Okano, Kenichiro. 1995b. "Traumatic mental disorders and their spectrums". *Japanese Journal of Psychiatric Treatment,* Vol. 10, No. 1: 9-19 (in Japanese)

[1997. *Japanese Journal of Psychiatric Treatment,* Vol. 12, No. 2].

CHAPTER 6

STUDY ON THE PATHOLOGICAL PERSONALITY IN THE OBJECT RELATION THEORY IN ENGLAND: ESPECIALLY ON THE CONCEPT OF THE PATHOLOGICAL ORGANIZATION

1. Introduction

In actual clinical practice, especially in the urban area, the number of outpatient visits and inpatient treatment of patients with classic schizophrenia and manic-depressive disorder have levelled off. However, medical consultation visits for adolescent problems (an indigenous group) and adult personality disorder (borderline, schizoid, narcissistic, etc.) are increasing. Schizophrenia and classical manic-depressive disorder have become milder and have become possible to be treated at the outpatient clinics, except in severe cases, due to the development of drug therapy.

Instead, corresponding to the so-called non-psychotic patient population described above is becoming an extremely urgent clinical challenge. The patient population includes male patients with "primary withdrawal", and female patients with emotionally unstable personality disorders associated with eating disorder, self-injurious behaviour, or suicide attempts, and, therapeutically, many of them require psychotherapy with a firm structure such as dynamic psychotherapy. This is especially true for psychiatric outpatients at university hospitals and general hospitals. At the outpatient clinic of the mental health and welfare centre where I work, we see many patients with personality disorders too.

Such non-psychiatric patients have long been placed in a slightly minor position in Japanese psychiatry, and even today, lectures of psychiatry for medical students focus on psychotic disorders. This is certainly applicable for psychiatric treatment in psychiatry-specialized hospitals which focus on the treatment of disorders such as schizophrenia. However, at medical sites centred on outpatient medical practice, such as the above-mentioned general hospitals and clinics in the urban areas, there is an increasing need for diagnostic methods and diagnostic criteria for personality disorders, and provision of psychoanalytical psychotherapy and other medical services.

The biggest obstacle is that, despite the rapid need for such medical services, medical insurance payment for psychiatric clinical practice is only one-third per working hour compared to that for clinical practice of other medical departments, and the payment standard of the medical insurance system is still centred on the treatment of disorders such as schizophrenia and manic-depressive states. Therefore, psychoanalytic psychotherapy, which requires much workforce and time, heads the list of unprofitable clinical practice. However, at clinical sites, a significant number of patients who require such treatment come for medical consultation. In Japan, which rapidly came to have a developed country-type urban culture, the system of insurance medical treatment points centred on developing-country-type mental disorders no longer can support the treatment system for patients with new types of developed-country-type non-psychotic disorders.

The diagnostic interviews for personality disorder are conducted for 50-minutes for 4 times. This diagnostic interview method is important for therapeutic judgement. Especially, if diagnosis is briefly conducted using a criterion such as DSM-IV, there is a possibility that patients with a background of high-functioning pervasive developmental disorder are mixed in patients diagnosed with personality disorder. It is necessary to be careful because patients with a background of high-functioning pervasive developmental disorder do not apply to psychoanalytical psychotherapy; supportive educational therapy and environmental therapy will be the main approaches for them. The author has participated in various case study meetings held all over Japan. Among the cases presented at those meetings, many patients with high-functioning pervasive developmental disorder were mixed up with the patients presented as intractable cases. Psychoanalytical psychotherapy requires a lot of time and workforce, so it is an important task to prevent the selection of inappropriate treatment cases by such initial inappropriate diagnoses.

In order to be able to make appropriate decisions, it is a prerequisite for a psychiatrist to first accumulate sufficient clinical experience with various types of patients with disorders such as schizophrenia, manic-depressive illness, and temperamental psychiatric illness, and then master psychoanalytical psychiatry.

2. Studies on pathological personality in object relation theory in the UK

"Pathological organization" proposed by J. Steiner, a Kleinian psychoanalyst, is a representative achievement of studies on pathological personality in contemporary UK. The British theory of object relations (in a broad sense) has two streams: the Kleinian school and the independent school. Since I, the author, have received much influence of the Kleinian school, I would like to mainly introduce the Kleinian theory. Here I will refer to the formation process of "pathological organization" in the history of the Kleinian school, and clarify its clinical significance.

(1) Klein's study on manic-depressive disorder and schizophrenia

Melanie Klein of the British Psychoanalytical Society revealed the early object relation of 0-year-old babies through psychoanalytic research of young children with severe neurosis or psychosis. Based on the clinical findings of psychoanalytic therapy in adult patients with manic-depressive disorder or schizophrenia, she proposed the developmental internal object relation theory of the depressive position (1935) and the paranoid-schizoid position (1946). This study, which is a study on psychosis and manic-depressive disorder, became the basis for later studies on various personality disorders.

a Paranoid-schizoid position

Although Klein proposed the paranoid-schizoid position later than the depressive position, I will first explain the period that is earlier in the development theory. The paranoid-schizoid position was proposed in 1946 and was studied until around 1960. It occupies a crucial position in psychoanalysis as an important early development theory and a pathology of schizophrenia, even in current times. This concept shows the early object relation, which was detected in the findings of psychoanalysis in children and in psychoanalytic therapy of adult patients with schizophrenia, and was clarified through the observation of the patients' primitive inner world and the transference to the therapist. Schizophrenia is thought to develop in cases when there is a conflicting hindrance in the development of early object relation and pathologically excessive anxiety is seen. In patients with schizophrenia, those primitive unresolved worlds of object relation remain split-off in their unconsciousness and are carried over unresolved until adulthood.

There is a normal "paranoid-schizoid position" in healthy children. When excessive anxiety is too strong, a state of pathological "paranoid-schizoid position" occurs, and if that state is split-off in the mind without being integrated, it becomes a predisposition for severe mental disorder such as adult schizophrenia. In this way, there are normal and pathological paranoid-schizoid positions, however, since Klein does not use terms that clearly distinguish those states, it has caused some confusion for readers. It was the study of "pathological organization" that clarified this confusion.

The "paranoid-schizoid position" represents the inner world of babies from birth to 4-5 months old. Such young babies live in a part object world where the mother's breast, face and other parts cannot be recognized as belongings to the same person's body. In that part object world, a temporal continuity is not established yet. The babies are terrified with annihilation anxiety and persecutory anxiety. They split and sort out part objects that give satisfaction to them (good objects) from bad objects that give frustration to them. They cannot recognize that they are experiences with the same mother (Splitting of good and bad objects).

When exposed to anxiety, babies cope with such anxiety experiences by trying to use primitive defence mechanisms such as splitting, projective identification, denial, and omnipotence.

Healthy children, under proper care from their mother, are less likely to be excessively exposed to intense anxiety and develop into the next step. On the other hand, when a baby is not constitutionally tolerant enough of anxiety or when the mother's care is inadequate, the baby is exposed to excessive annihilation anxiety and persecutory anxiety, and a pathological "paranoid-schizoid position" is formed because the vulnerable self cannot cope with them. If it is split-off and remains unresolved in the unconsciousness, it forms a predisposition that causes disorders such as schizophrenia and paranoia after adolescence.

b Depressive position

The depressive position was studied and clarified by Klein from 1935 to around 1940 before the above-mentioned paranoid-schizoid position, and is based on the findings obtained through the treatment of adult manic-depressive disorder. It is the basic pathology of psychogenic manic-depressive disorder even in modern times.

At 5 to 6 months of age, babies come to be able to recognize that the good and bad objects in the paranoid-schizoid position are experiences with the same mother. In other words, babies begin to notice that the objects that are their most beloved ideal good objects and the bad objects that cause them frustration actually belong to the same mother. At that time, the babies come to experience abandonment anxiety and a strong sense of guilt (depressive anxiety). Then, they begin to show "concern" that they might have hurt the object by their own aggression and possess a "feeling of reparation". This is the first period when the personality integrates and babies feel their ambivalent first depressive conflict.

Babies who have a well-internalized satisfactory object relation before this time can overcome the challenges of this depressive position and can grow further on. Conversely, when the experience of frustration is excessive and the conflict is too strong, a pathological depressive position is formed without the conflict being dealt with. It is split-off in the mind and persists, and later becomes a predisposition for disorders such as manic-depressive illness.

(2) W. Bion's study on psychotic personality and non-psychotic personality

Through the 1950s and 1960s, Bion enthusiastically conducted psychoanalytic research on schizophrenia, being influenced by the study of Klein's paranoid-schizoid position. He not only confirmed that the patients with schizophrenia had a pathology of the paranoid-schizoid position, but also further clarified the process of formation of their psychotic situation. He proposed that a "psychotic personality" that presents a pathological situation of such paranoid-schizoid position exists in the mind as a partial self.

Bion also considered that any individual with a psychotic personality always has a non-psychotic personality part and there exists a power in them to build a therapeutic relationship with the therapist.

(3) H. Rosenfeld's study on schizophrenia and destructive narcissistic organization

Rosenfeld, along with Bion, H. Segal and others, cooperated with Klein and diligently practiced psychoanalytic therapy for patients with schizophrenia from the 1940s to 1960s, and generated many clinical outcomes. In addition, he studied difficult-to-treat cases of non-psychotic pathological personalities from the 1960s to the 1970s; that includes patients with drug addiction, sexual perversion, severe hypochondria, and emotionally unstable personality. This is a representative study of pathological personalities in the United Kingdom.

He focused on the patients who developed a so-called negative therapeutic reaction in psychoanalytic therapy of such patients. In other words, he focused on the patients who, during the course of treatment, showed intense acting-outs including violence or self-injurious behaviour, antisocial behaviour, suicide attempts, and caused sudden interruptions by devaluing treatment; and clarified the pathology of the inner world. Rosenfeld then revealed that such patients unconsciously had a self-destructive destructive narcissistic organization in their unconsciousness. He considered understanding and interpretation of the trend were extremely essential for clinical practice. This has become representative research on borderline cases in the United Kingdom.

This destructive narcissistic organization is a part self, which is formed when the self incorporates an aggressive object and identifies with it. The self extremely idealizes the part of self that has such a destructive tendency. Since the self idealizes the part of the destructive self, it actively attacks the various creative and developmental possibilities of other parts of self. Phenomenally, it looks like sadism or masochism. The aggressive part of self actively attacks and destroys the other parts of self when they trust the object or healthily depend on it and try to start growing. It is a state where the relation between the original aggressive destructive object and the individual is internalized intact and iterated in the inner world. The individual creates a pathological part of his/her self using the internalized destructive object that most afflicted him/herself as a material, and identifies with and idealizes it. He/she then begins to enthusiastically attack the other normal parts of self.

The patient has a tendency to identify with the object which once attacked him/her, and attack him/herself and abandon all possibilities. It is important for the therapist to make this tendency clear and work it through. This pathological personality theory had a great influence on the following Steiner's study on "pathological organization".

(4) Steiner's study on pathological organization

Based on the above research, John Steiner clarified the internal structure of pathological personality from the 1980s to the 1990s. It was a developmental integration of the above stated perspectives of Klein, Bion and Rosenfeld. It can be said that the internal structural theory of the British pathological personality is completed for the time being.

The basic idea of Steiner's pathological organization is as follows:

(1) Patients with pathological personality present states including therapeutically awkward resistive states, negative therapeutic reactions, and destructive resistive states. The patients' pathological organization is related to this. That is, such patients constitute an organization consisting of pathological object relations in a part of their unconsciousness. It has a broad spectrum of aspects such as psychotic, manic-depressive, emotionally unstable, schizoid, narcissistic, and neurotic aspects.

(2) The beginning and formation process of this pathological organization is associated with early object relation. Steiner states that this pathological organization constitutes a pathological third position that deviates from the healthy developmental line of healthy paranoid-schizoid position and depressive position; and is positioned at the boundary between these two positions. The pathological organization stubbornly resists change, and its characteristics are perversion of object relations and addiction.

(3) The formation process is as follows: The baby forms a bad object by projectively identifying with the object that causes frustration and a part of self to the outside world. In order to secure its self from anxiety such as persecutory anxiety and abandonment anxiety against the bad object, the baby introjects the bad object into the self again and identifies with it (introjective identification) to form a pathological organization complex. It has a persecutory and depressive characteristic, typically with a part object relation tendency and a fluctuant tendency of integration, because it is made of an originally aggressive object, an amalgamation of selves.

Primitive defence mechanisms such as splitting, projective identification, and denial are active there. In the course of treatment, such pathological object relations are transferred to the therapist and cause acting-out.

(4) This pathological organization has various characteristics depending on the features of the object, the group of selves, that caused the frustration, and it shows versatile aspects of internal object relation; that is, from an aspect where the pathological disposition of early paranoid-schizoid position is central, to an aspect where excessive abandonment anxiety of the depressive position is prominent, and up to an aspect which has neurotic conflicts such as mourning.

(5) If those aspects are so strong that they dominate the self, they clinically appear as various personality disorders: for example, psychotic personality disorder, depressive personality disorder, schizoid personality disorder, borderline personality disorder and narcissistic personality disorder.

(6) Steiner subdivided the developmental stages to the paranoid-schizoid position and depressive position into four stages to organize them theoretically. He placed the characteristics of pathological organization corresponding to those developmental stages. (**Figure 1**)

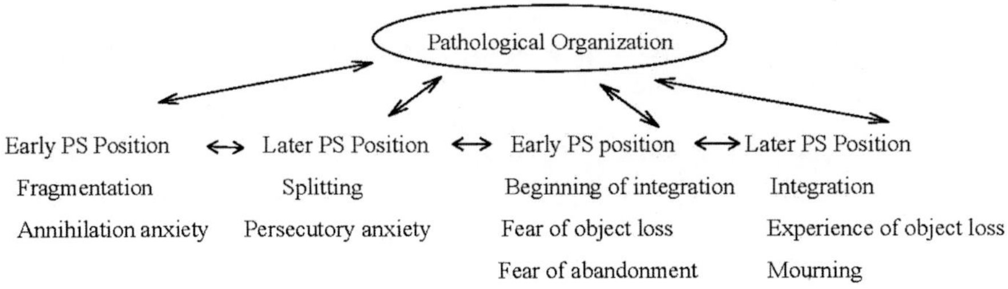

Figure 1. Paranoid-schizoid (PS) position and depressive (D) position

a Early paranoid-schizoid position

The early paranoid-schizoid position is characterized by annihilation anxiety. Normal babies experience a mild one, too, and their good object relations are sufficient and their anxiety is not so strong. In pathological cases, a pathological organization is formed in the self. Pathological organization principally involves annihilation fears of self and object, and is featured by primitive defence mechanisms (e.g., splitting, projective identification, etc.) and fragmentation. Steiner proposed a psychotic pathological organization with characteristic part object relations in this way. In such cases, severe schizophrenia develops in adulthood.

b Later paranoid-schizoid position

In the later paranoid-schizoid position, persecutory anxiety is characteristic. Individuals who encounter frustration at that period feature persecutory anxiety, primitive defence mechanisms including not-so-much severe splitting and projective identification, and slightly relieved part object relations.

If the object relations are filled with excessive anxiety at this period, a characteristic psychotic pathological organization is formed. If the problems of this period persist, disorders including schizophrenia, which claims adult persecutory anxiety, can be seen.

c Early depressive position

The early depressive position is a state in which integration and dismantling are fluctuant, and is characterized by fear of abandonment. Splitting and projective identification are relieved but are actively in action. Additionally, "introjection" becomes active and "manic defence" comes into appearance. When exposed to excessive anxiety, pathological organizations founded on pathological abandonment anxiety are formed. Clinically, they are personality disorders such as depressive personality disorder, borderline personality disorder, schizoid personality disorder, and narcissistic personality disorder.

d Later depressive position

Later depressive position is characterized by mourning of object loss and mourning work. Neurotic defences such as repression, projection, and displacement will appear. In pathological situations, neuroses such as obsessive-compulsive neurosis and hysteria will occur.

3. Case report

Here, I would like to introduce a case patient of severe borderline personality disorder, who was understood based on Steiner's concept of pathological organization.

(1) Patient

The patient was a 20-year-old woman. Her chief complaints included depersonalization, depressive attacks, overeating, and sense of self-insufficiency; and she could not tell what kind of person she was (identity disorder). Physically, she had severe pain and sense of stiffness all over her body. In addition, she had repeated suicide attempts by overdosing.

The patient was brought up strictly by her parents from infancy. Her mother prohibited her from leaving the study room, and forced her to study. Her father, who had intense emotional instability, hurled abusive language, and violently attacked the patient and her mother every day. The mother was selfish and although she was obedient to her violent husband, she was harsh to the patient and forced the patient to obey her: she was an overly education-minded mother. The patient had lived with fear towards her father since childhood. Superficially, the patient was docile, and she studied hard and her grades were excellent. Although she was bullied and isolated in her junior high school days, she continued to attend school.

(2) Therapeutic course

The patient was diagnosed and assessed to be eligible for psychoanalytic psychotherapy, and therapy was started once a week, at first. However, the patient repeatedly overdosed, became excited, and damaged properties at home, therefore, the therapist recommended hospitalization. Nevertheless, neither the family nor the patient herself accepted hospitalization, so it was decided that the patient would continue therapy as an outpatient. Although highly analgesic antipsychotics and anxiolytics were administered to somehow settle her violent acting-outs and emotional flooding, she did not calm down much. For outpatient care, patients with such repeated violent acting-outs and suicide attempts can sometimes be tranquilized by frequent psychoanalytic psychotherapy. Therefore, the therapist decided to conduct psychoanalytic therapy four times a week.

In the first month after the patient started to receive frequent therapy, she did not conduct any violent acting-outs or suicide attempts, and she came to be able to verbally express her experiences and use her thoughts.

The patient said that she had iterated traumatic relationships with men. The man she met when she joined the company she worked for was aggressive and violent. He demanded absolute obedience from the patient, and had sexual sadism. The patient could not escape, and, inside, she was full of fear.

At that time, since the fear of the patient when she met the male therapist was also reflected, the therapist interpreted that the patient had suspicion and fear against the therapist.

Additionally, the patient began to tell that her father was a fearsome person who had used violence against her mother, beat the patient, and ranted at them from when the patient was little. When the patient had hard feelings towards her father, even in the slightest terms, her whole body became stiff and strong pain occurred all over her whole body during therapy. After she left the therapy room, she would be overcome with a feeling of isolation and fear along with a strong sense of guilt, which caused persecutory anxiety. For example, she became scared of people's eyes or felt that the surrounding buildings would fall over and attack her on her way home. In addition, depersonalization and dissociative symptoms appeared, and her overeating became severe. Nevertheless, the patient came to therapy without skipping.

The patient's relationship with her boyfriend during this period was perversive. The patient was intuitively strongly attracted to a man who had a violent aspect of her father, and got embroiled in a sado-masochistic world. In fact, during sexual intercourses with her boyfriend, he injured the patient's body. The patient formed a fused world with the man, and tried to live completely obediently in the man's world negating her own spontaneous feelings and intentions. She denied that she was hurt and suffering, but as the therapist interpreted in therapy that she was hurt, she realized her discomfort and disgust towards the man. She then developed severe depression, fear of abandonment and a strong sense of guilt. The patient also became emotionally confused when she thought she was rejected by the man even in the slightest way, and she harmed herself and took overdoses. This is a masochistic, perversive personality type of pathological organization.

The patient gradually came to realize that she had been completely submissive to her parents, especially her father, and had lived as much as possible in the world of her father's intentions, splitting-off her critical feelings and spontaneity. After the therapist arduously interpreted this, the patient began to recall her complex emotions towards her father who repeatedly abused her, and her mother who stayed on his side without helping the patient. Then, as the patient returned home after treatment, an explosive anger towards her parents surged up, however, at the same time, dissociative symptoms appeared, and the patient did not have any memories of that period.

The therapist decided to discuss with the patient why she continued to have a strong interest and dependence on her father and men whom she most feared and disliked. As a result, she gradually became aware of the paradoxical unnaturalness of herself being obediently devoted to her father, whom she most feared and was hurt by, and men who resembled him, while possessing a strong sense of guilt. She came to realize that she also had strong hatred and aggression, too. At that time, the patient developed depressive attacks, and had severe systemic pain and depersonalization.

The therapist was highly idealized, but when the therapist took a vacation or interpreted the patient's fear and masochistic attitude towards the therapist, her rage against the man and anger against her father became more intense and she began to show violent acting-outs.

The therapist patiently gave interpretations to the patient who repeated such acting-outs and iterated ambivalent and contradictory object relations, so that the patient could promote her self-understanding.

The therapist often asked the patient why she was so strongly interested in such destructive men and father and whether she was aware of the contradiction. The patient answered that she was attracted to such terrible men without knowing why. She continued that ordinary kind men have no presence, their presence was as faint as shadows, and she could not be attracted to them as a male. The therapist also discussed the issue that the patient considered that the therapist was a good person but had no presence like them, so the therapeutic experience itself was diluted.

Additionally, the following issues were discussed: i) When the patient approached such sadistic men, she would exclude her fears and disgusts and make them perversive to be attracted to aggressive men. ii) When the patient did not obey such destructive men, an intense abandonment experience and a sense of guilt arose, and she would not try to leave them. This also showed the intensity of the patient's painful and hurt experience, which has remained unresolved in her mind. iii) For the patient, a person who tried to support and help her, such as the therapist, had become nothing more than a helpless and faint presence, so, after all, the patient gained a false feeling of security under such destructive men. The patient came to understand such things.

The patient said, "I have started to feel critical about my father and boyfriend, but at that time a strong fear of isolation arises and I begin to feel fear that I will become completely lonely in this whole world. So, I try not to feel them and rush and go back to my father or boyfriend."

The patient recalled many of her parents' aggressive, hurtful, and violent worlds, but after that, she repeatedly had strong physical pain and intense fear. The therapist interpreted that behind her clinging-on to her parents who hurt her so much and intense guilt towards them, there conversely existed fierce hatred and aggression towards such parents.

The patient had felt that it was her mission to act as an intermediary for her parents from long ago, and she recalled like a flashback the scenes where her mother and herself were violently abused; and repeatedly had extreme fear and sobbed terribly. When the patient was with the therapist, these experiences became clear and she would become upset and guilty, but when she left the interview room, her memories of what she had said would fade and she just continued to feel isolated or depressed. Then she would have a conflictive feeling and tried to return to her parents and boyfriend.

During this period, the therapist continued to have an overwhelming sense of fear (a counter-transference) in the patient's destructive world and the world of intense guilt and strong clinging-on. This also seemed to be related to the fact that the patient herself had destructiveness and aggression which were beyond her control.

Eventually, symptoms such as self-injurious behaviour, depersonalization, dissociation, and overeating disappeared, and the patient regained her spontaneous world, which she had split-off.

However, this was something that was even more painful for the patient. The patient met another man and fell into a sadistic relationship. She had unconsciously chosen a man who also had a violent and sadistic tendency, again. The therapist patiently interpreted the patient's issue of choosing such a pathological object in association to her ambivalent relationship with her father. In the midst of a conflict between such a man and intense abandonment anxiety and feeling of guilt, she then fell into a transient psychotic state, when she finally was going to separate with the man.

Even so, the patient came to recognize how contradictory and how harmful and painful her experiences and actions were, and how tremendous the anger and resentment she had were. At such times, the patient shared her injurious experiences sobbing and shedding buckets of tears.

The patient gradually became aware of her pathological world of repetition compulsion and came to realize how she had suffered from the abusive relationship with her father, and how she was terribly confused because, although she had tried to save her mother from the violence, her mother was always on her father's side.

The patient is in a state where an unresolved pathology from the later paranoid schizoid position to the early depressive position, which is filled with persecutory fear, fear of abandonment and a strong sense of guilt towards the violent world, continues to exist in her personality. Although it presents an emotionally confused state, it is stable as a pathological organization. It is filled with addiction and perversion, and exhibits strong resistance to change. It also has a great influence on the formation of the patient's clinical picture as a patient with borderline personality disorder.

4. Conclusion

I explained the formation process of Steiner's "pathological organization", which is a typical pathological personality theory of the Kleinians in England. I then introduced a case of severely emotionally unstable personality disorder and showed that the pathological organization proposed by Steiner was strongly active.

In psychoanalysis, the therapeutic structure is strictly adhered to, and a therapeutic approach is taken by giving interpretations centred on transference and countertransference based on free association. This personality theory was formed based on the multi-layered data obtained by such a setting.

References

(1) Bion, Wilfred Ruprecht. 1967. *Second Thoughts*. London: Heinemann.

(2) Klein, Melanie. 1935/1975. "A Contribution to the Psychogenesis of Manic-Depressive States". In *The Writings of Melanie Klein*, Vol. 1: 262-289. London: Hogarth Press.

(3) Klein, Melanie. 1940/1975. "Mourning and Its Relation to Manic-Depressive States". In *The Writings of Melanie Klein*, Vol. 1: 344-369. London: Hogarth Press.

(4) Klein, Melanie. 1946/1975. "Notes on Some Schizoid Mechanisms". In *The Writings of Melanie Klein*, Vol. 3: 1-24. London: Hogarth Press.

(5) Rosenfeld, Herbert. 1965. *Psychotic States*, London: Hogarth Press.

(6) Rosenfeld, Herbert. 1971. "A Clinical Approach to the Psychoanalytic Theory of the Life and Death Instincts: An Investigation into the Aggressive Aspects of Narcissism". *International Journal of Psychoanalysis*, 52: 169-178.

(7) Steiner, John. 1993. *Psychic Retreats: Pathological Organizations in Psychotic, Neurotic and Borderline Patients*. London: Hogarth.

[2003, *Japanese Journal of Psychopathology*. Vol. 24, No. 2.]

CHAPTER 7

PSYCHOANALYTIC STUDIES ON PSYCHOTIC PERSONALITY DISORDER, AND ITS OVERVIEW: THROUGH STUDIES ON SCHIZOPHRENIA

1. Introduction

This paper features the studies regarding psychoanalytic approaches for "psychotic personality". Historically, they have been conducted as studies on schizophrenia, so the approaches will be summarized here as the history of studies on schizophrenia. S. Freud discussed psychosis including schizophrenia and manic depression, and considered that manic depression was also not a target for psychoanalytic treatment. In this paper, the term psychosis is used for a group of patients with schizophrenia or schizophrenia-like illnesses. In recent years, it is considered that there are subgroups in such schizophrenic patients: patients with psychogenic schizophrenia, in which the problem of early object relations is the mainstream, and patients with schizophrenia who have a stronger biophysiological predisposition. Psychoanalytic approach is indicated for the former psychogenic schizophrenia. More recently, in my experience, it is known that there are patients with a schizophrenia-like illness with a background of high-functioning pervasive developmental disorder whose intellectual level is normal or higher, and in such cases, the developmental therapy becomes the main approach.

Historically, S. Freud believed that patients with schizophrenia were unable to develop transferences because they were regressed into an objectless world of narcissism, thus were not subject to psychoanalysis. The only case of schizophrenia he gave a consideration to was the Schreber case. However, he did not directly treat the patient, but just gave a psychoanalytical consideration on an autobiography on psychosis published by the patient himself. There, S. Freud focused on the patient's world of part-object relation and mechanism of projection. However. he did not consider that schizophrenia was subject to psychoanalytic treatment. He thought that when taking a psychotherapeutic approach, the technique should be modified. Although they were critical about this Freud's idea, analysts who basically took on this way of thinking were mainly American ego psychologists and American Neo-Freudians including P. Federn, H. Sullivan, E. From-Reichman, and H. Searles.

M. Klein criticized S. Freud's theory of narcissism, and considered that the state of narcissism was not an objectless world, as S. Freud thought, but actually a state of an early primitive internal object relation, and discovered that object relations existed from immediately after birth. Klein stated that schizophrenic patients were fixed in a state where they were introverted in such an internal object relation, clinically presenting psychotic transferences and transferring such primitive object relation to the therapist. She also said that the therapist could deal with transferences by interpreting them. In 1946, M. Klein theorized the world of such primitive object relations as the "paranoid-schizoid position". Around the time Klein presented this concept, Kleinian analysts began to treat schizophrenic patients with psychoanalysis. In particular, energetic researches were carried out mainly by H. Segal, H. Rosenfeld, and W. Bion, who directly received guidance from M. Klein. What was characteristic was that even in the treatment for schizophrenia, they adhered to the setting of 50 minutes, 5 to 6 times a week, focused on transference interpretations, and did not try to adopt techniques which promoted supportive techniques and positive transferences. In their researches, they discovered psychotic transference, and found that patients with schizophrenia could develop transferences and had a possibility of being eligible for psychoanalytic treatment and understanding.

In this paper, I would like to give an overview on these two major trends regarding studies on schizophrenia.

2. S. Freud's Theory on Psychosis

Freud himself discussed psychosis including both schizophrenia and manic-depressive illness, but here I would like to primarily share his views on schizophrenia. Freud was negative about applying psychoanalysis to schizophrenia, and when indicating it for patients with schizophrenia, he considered that the technique should be modified to a supportive approach since patients were incapable of developing transferences. This Freud's way of thinking has had a great influence on his subsequent approach to psychosis in psychoanalysis.

Despite that, Freud has a keen interest in psychosis and made some important considerations, some of which have become the basic perspectives of subsequent studies on psychosis.

(1) The novel "*Gradiva*"

In 1907, S. Freud analysed the dream of the main character in the literary work "Gradiva", who was in a delusional state, and presented his lover's function as a therapist in the process of the recovery of the main character's health ("Delusions and Dreams in Jansen's "Gradiva"": 1907). The male protagonist has a so-called schizoid personality tendency, tends to be withdrawn, and is absorbed in biology. He falls in love with a Roman woman sculpture and becomes paranoidly convinced that she had died in the tragedy of Pompei. He actually goes to the ruins of Pompei and tries to meet her. The sculpture woman appears in his dream, and even after he awakens, he confuses the dream with the reality. Then, his professor's daughter, whom he actually was deeply in love with, comes to study the ruins of Pompei as an archaeologist, and meets the main character. He confuses her, a real woman, with Gradiva and responds in a delusional world. He also experiences an auditory hallucination that the buzzing of flies was a conversation between lovers. The real woman who saw this situation understood that he was in a delusional state and makes every effort hoping that he would return to the real world. She does not immediately deny his delusional world, and acts his delusional world together with him by entering into his omnipotent world and fulfilling his demands. She gradually succeeds in bringing him back to the real world. The man becomes aware of his repressed sexual world and realizes that it was actually the real woman that he had been seeking for and had been in love with. Becoming aware of that, he escapes from the delusional world.

Freud stated that the way that the real woman satisfied the patient's omnipotence and gradually brought him back to the real world was equivalent to the technique of psychoanalytic therapy for patients in delusional states, except that psychoanalysts maintain their neutrality and discretion and never fall into a personal relationship with the patient. Here Freud emphasized the content of the dreams and delusional experiences of the patients who are in a delusional state, and considered that the treatment would be psychoanalysis where the analyst would lead the patient to become conscious of what they had been repressing. It is mysterious why Freud did not later clinically develop this therapeutic theory. However, this was a perspective which was developed later on in the treatment for psychosis by P. Federn, E. From-Reichman, H. Sullivan, H. Searles and other analysts. I wonder why successive researchers have not mentioned "Gradiva" regarding Freud's view on the treatment for delusional psychosis.

This Freud's paper on Gradiva is also a forerunner of a technical theory as a literature theory which analyses the novel's story itself. Additionally, through the analyses of the two important dreams that are told in the story,

Freud brilliantly analyses that there exists the protagonist's repressed sexual world where he seeks a woman in the background of this story. Freud admired the overwhelming power of the author's creativity and imagination. S. Freud had a complex towards artists all his life long.

(2) The Schreber case (1911)

Although Freud thought that psychoanalytic therapy was not applicable for schizophrenia, he was keenly interested in its pathology. Especially, at that time, analysts of the Zurich school such as E. Bleuler, G. Jung, and K. Abraham were ahead in the study of schizophrenia, and he must have had a sense of competitiveness towards them.

Schreber, a person with schizophrenia who was well-known at the time, published a memoir of his accusation to the court when he was forced to be admitted to a mental hospital. It was a detailed record of the delusional world of psychosis. Psychiatrists at the time made various comments on it. Freud also paid attention to the memoir and made a pathological consideration on schizophrenia. However, this was not a therapeutic case report but a consideration on psychoanalytic pathology based on a memoir published by a patient himself.

The description of the memoir revealed that Schreber had developed a delusional transference to his analyst, Flechsig, and S. Freud considered that it was a homosexual transference. He believed that the projection of this homosexual libido and the transformation of meanings were important factors in the formation of delusions. Flechsig, Schreber's treating psychiatrist, appeared as a major object along with God in Schreber's delusional world. Freud stated that the delusions including the delusion where Schreber turns into a woman and has sexual intercourse with God, the delusion where Flechsig exists in split entities, the delusion where God is distinguished by the upper and lower, front and back were related to the homosexual complex against his father and brother, and those complexes were "transferred" to his analyst, Flechsig. This is inconsistent with Freud's claim that patients with schizophrenia do not develop "transferences". Freud also stated that the mechanism of projection played a major role in the symptomatic phenomena seen there.

In such way, Freud admits that Schreber had developed transferences to his analyst, although they were delusional. Nevertheless, Freud was negative about the therapeutic potential of applying psychoanalysis to schizophrenia.

(3) The pleasure/unpleasure principle and reality principle: the two mental principles

Here, Freud describes the state of primary narcissism by comparing it to a chicken egg (Formulations on the Two Principles of Mental Functioning). Babies are in the primary thinking process based on the pleasure/unpleasure principle. When they need an object in the outside world, they hallucinatorily obtain what they want so that they can be satisfied for a while. However, if their need is still not fulfilled, they have no other choice but to require an external object and come to live in a world of the reality principle. That is a world of the secondary thinking process, and the babies will need to adapt to the external reality through their sensory organs, consciousness, attention, memorization, memories, thoughts and actions. Fread also revealed that thought is a process of experimental actions of internal trials and verification. Still, in a repressed and unconscious world, the primary thinking process is still active. Although in schizophrenia, the secondary thinking process is often impaired, Freud did not develop this issue any further. Bion, W. took up the issue of the impaired secondary thinking process in his study on psychotic personality in the 1950s. This paper provided the basic perspectives.

(4) On narcissism (1914)

Freud stated in the first part of his paper on narcissism ("On Narcissism": 1914) that the narcissism theory is primarily aimed at explaining autism in schizophrenia. He considered that schizophrenia could not be explained without considering the ego-preservative instinct. He also said that such patients are in a narcissistic state and therefore cannot develop transferences. For this reason, Freud called schizophrenia and manic-depressive disorder as narcissistic neuroses, and on the other hand, called hysteria and obsessive-compulsive disorder, which can develop transferences, as transference neuroses.

According to Freud, newborn babies feel everything is satisfied and they are in a state where they cannot recognize objects. All libidos are directed towards the ego and new born babies are in a complete self-sufficient state. S. Freud called this as primary narcissism. When the babies begin to experience hunger and frustration, they seek an object for the first time and become aware of its existence for the first time. They begin to cathect libido to the object. This is the beginning of the involvement with objects. Schizophrenia is a state where an individual, when exposed to some frustration, withdraws all libido for the object (decathexis) and directs the libido toward the ego. Freud regarded this as a state of narcissism.

In any case, an individual who has withdrawn all libido from the object cannot have an object relation because he/she cathects all his/her libido to his/her ego. Since this state is similar to the state of primary narcissism, S. Freud called it as secondary narcissism. This group of patients with schizophrenia, who are in secondary narcissism, cannot develop transferences to the therapist, thus Freud considered that they were not eligible for psychoanalytic treatment. However, he stated that since only part of the mind of patients with schizophrenia is decathected, the healthy part is functioning. If so, that healthy part should be capable of developing transferences, however, it seems that Freud considered that the healthy part was just a part that would cooperate with treatment.

Consideration on schizophrenia becomes eclipsed in the middle of this paper on narcissism. The argument proceeds to the narcissistic object choice seen in normal psychology and how the parents' narcissistic relation to their babies are. Freud emphasizes that, finally, a unique ego-ideal world to satisfy narcissism is built in the mind. This paper was a forerunner of the later studies on the formation of super-ego. There, the issue of schizophrenia is not discussed much. However, it implies the process of introjecting the image of the object together when the libido is withdrawn from the object. Freud later clarified the issue in his paper, "Mourning and Melancholia" (1917). He took up the issue of introjection and identification of lost objects in manic-depressive illness, and was in the process of clarifying the formation process of internal objects. It is strange that he did not try to consider schizophrenia in the same way. This was later clarified by M. Klein as the formation process of internal object relations in infants, and as the role of internal object relations in schizophrenia.

3. K. Abraham's study

Abraham worked on schizophrenia with Bleuler and Jung from the 1900s as a Zurich school analyst, conducted a joint study with Freud and became his leading disciple. Since Abraham was a Jew, it was impossible for him to get a key job at a university, thus he opened a clinic in Berlin in 1911 and operated a psychoanalytic research institute and a psychiatric ward. Abraham energetically conducted psychoanalytic treatment and research for manic depressive illness, which Freud believed was not an indication for psychoanalysis at the time. Abraham advocated that the ambivalent fixation status in the early and late anal stages, in which patient have a 6-month-old disposition, is the origin of the pathology of manic depression. He implied that schizophrenia was associated with the babies' fixation to the oral phase, suggesting that it could be treated by psychoanalysis. The well-known theory on development which Abraham presented at the time was based on S. Freud's theory, but more detailed. He stated that part objects, ambivalence, and early development of 0-year-olds are important, which had a great influence on Klein's theory. Abraham stated that, in the treatment of manic-depressive illness, patients develop transferences of early development, and demonstrated that therapeutic results could be achieved if the therapist interprets the transferences while maintaining the therapist's neutrality. Freud felt that his claim was not accepted and his theory was overturned thus expressed his displeasure, however, he later made a pathological consideration on manic-depressive illness in his paper "Mourning and Melancholia" and accepted a part of Abraham's research.

What is important is that M. Klein, who later developed a ground-breaking pathology and therapeutic theory for schizophrenia, stayed in Berlin from 1921 to 1926 and received Abraham's guidance and training analysis. In Berlin, Abraham recommended Klein to treat very young, severely ill children aged 2 to 3, and she gained a lot of revolutionary insights. Freud said at this time, too, that children under the age of 3 would not be eligible for psychoanalytic therapy because an inner world has not been built in them and they cannot give free associations since they do not have an ability to express themselves linguistically. In a letter to Abraham, Freud ordered him to immediately stop Klein's clinical activities, but Abraham rejected the instruction saying that Klein's research would be a revolution in psychoanalysis. As shown below, this became a major turning point for this study to develop into the contemporary object relation theory and Kleinian theory.

4. P. Federn's Study

Federn (1871-1950) has been introduced to Japan in details by Dr. Keigo Okonogi. Federn criticized Freud's theory of narcissistic neurosis, advocating that even psychotic patients can develop transferences and a psychotherapeutic approach is possible towards them.

(1) Theory of schizophrenia

Federn considered that an important pathology of schizophrenia lies in the vulnerability of its ego boundary. He placed importance on ego-feelings. He stated that individuals can feel what is related to ego-feelings by which they can have subjective emotions as the inside of their selves, and on the other hand, consider experiences unrelated to ego-feelings as external experiences. In this way, individuals distinguish between their internal experiences and external experiences. This ego boundary functions properly in healthy individuals. However, if the ego-feelings become vulnerable in the process of psychosis, the individuals come to have experiences where the unconscious world enters the ego, or even the experience of the external world enters the ego. For individuals, since both of them do not accompany any ego-feelings, they are experienced as external worlds. Therefore, protrusions of the self's unconscious experiences are experienced as delusion or hallucination experiences, or something that are occurring in the external world, and are mixed up with the outside world. In other words, as a result of the vulnerability of the ego boundary, discriminability between thought (idea) and objects is impaired; an incorrect sense of reality of thought (idea) is acquired, and incorrect conviction (certainty) of judgment or reasoning and actions accompanying it occur. This is the basic core of the pathology of schizophrenia. The goal for Federn's psychotherapy was to fix the vulnerability of this ego boundary.

(2) Federn's therapeutic theory and therapeutic techniques

Federn had the following three points as his basic perspective. First, psychotic patients have an ability to develop transferences. Secondly, since healthy parts remain in the ego and not all parts are damaged, the healthy part of the ego can obtain self-understanding for the pathological part of the ego. Thirdly, a part of the ego maintains health and can interact with the reality of the outside world. Based on these basic perspectives, Federn considered that psychoanalytic assistance is possible for psychotic patients.

Since patients with schizophrenia lose ego cathexis, their ego boundary becomes vulnerable. Thus, Federn's therapeutic goal was to recover that ego cathexis. In order to reconstruct the internal ego boundary, the goal is to obtain a dynamic and energy-economic equilibrium between the unconscious drive (id) or the protruding force of the past infantile ego state and the ego. For that purpose, the ego will be supported to enhance its suppression towards the id. In order to reconstruct the external ego boundary, the ego's reality testing ability and function for thoughts will be supported to enhance the learning ability of the ego function. As the ego cathexis is recovered and the ego boundary is reconstructed, the adult ego state can dominate the infantile ego state and they become re-integrated.

On this account, Federn corrected the psychoanalytic techniques as follows. First of all, he abandoned free association. This is because he considered that becoming conscious of the unconscious drive and the state of the infantile ego through free-association would promote the pathological process and be dangerous since patients are already excessively conscious of them due to the vulnerability of their ego boundary. Secondly, Federn considered that positive transferences should be promoted and not be analysed. He believed that maintaining positive transferences would promote ego cathexis and was important for the reconstruction of the ego boundary. Federn considered that a genuine absolute mother-like existence who could omnipotently fulfil the patient's ego requirements was necessary as a therapeutic partner. Actually, a nurse, Gertrud Schwing, worked as an important therapeutic partner for Federn.

This Federn's research had a major impact on the American therapists who have been working on psychoanalytic therapy for patients with schizophrenia, such as Sullivan, From-Reichman, and Searles.

5. Studies on Schizophrenia in the United States

(1) H. Sullivan

Sullivan (1892–1948) energetically focused on the treatment for schizophrenia. He considered that the origin of the pathology of schizophrenia was in the relationship between the baby and the mother. He established a special hospital ward and treated patients with schizophrenia based on support by a group of analysts of the same sex as the patient. He stated that it was important that the staff does not refute the patient's delusional misperceptions, but tries to understand them as much as possible. It is reminiscent of what Freud said in his paper on "Gradiva". Such environmental support becomes the basis of the psychoanalytic approach, and when a certain period of time passes, there comes a time when the patient becomes able to accept a psychoanalytic approach. When the time came, Sullivan revealed the patient's forgotten personal history and took a psychoanalytic approach with a goal of reconstructing the true chronology of the psychosis. He also placed importance on positive transferences and tried not to deal with negative transferences. He listed staff and therapists who he considered unsuitable for the psychotherapeutic approach for patients with schizophrenia as follows: (1) those who are of the opposite sex to the patient; (2) psychiatrists who have not received training analysis or have just recently received it; (3) those who are philosophical and over-thinking; (4) resistant homosexuals; (5) ideal reformers; (6) psychiatrists who are strongly oriented toward power and principalities over their fellows; (7) some priests, etc.

(2) F. Fromm-Reichman

Fromm-Reichmann (1890–1957) also worked earnestly on schizophrenia, but was critical of Federn's and other analysts' approach, which sought to establish a borderless relationship with the therapist which is like an absolute mother's care. She believed that that the therapist should hold his/her neutrality, and it was therapeutically important for the therapist to maintain essential therapeutic positive transferences with an appropriate approach and not to deal with negative emotions.

Fromm-Reichman considered that patients with schizophrenia had severe traumatic experiences early in development. Later, she came to argue that transference analysis, which she previously strongly criticized, should be conducted. She came to state that patients have fear of approaching their dependent objects and problems of hidden anger and that they should be interpreted. However, in order for patients to understand the dynamics, she used much guidance and instructions.

(3) H. Searles

H. Searles (1918-2015) worked most vigorously on the treatment of schizophrenia in contemporary United States. He conformed to M. Mahler's development theory, and as for schizophrenia, Searles considered schizophrenic patients were individuals who are fixated in the stages of what Marler called the autism phase and symbiosis phase. Also, the transferences of such patients are extremely primitive ego organizations and are comparable to those of infants living in a part-object world.

His therapeutic techniques are as follows: (1) The therapist aims to build a symbiotic relationship with the patient, and the patient aims to separate and become independent from this symbiotic world. (2) Verbal interpretation is contraindicated and the patient is in a state where he/she cannot adopt verbal communication well. The patient uses the therapist as his/her own ego and transfers a diverse part-object world to the therapist. The therapist needs an ability to be able to endure and even enjoy it. (So-called "co-psychotic therapy"). At this time, the patient's ego is enhanced through identification with the therapist. In this symbiotic stage, the patient experiences a part of him/herself as an object. Searles did not make statements on splitting of ego or self, or about concrete thinking, but he had often described such phenomena in his clinical records.

Nevertheless, Searles regarded symbiotic transferences as interdependent and told his patients about his own affection and hatred. H. Rosenfeld criticized that this was a big mistake and said Searles was not treating countertransference appropriately and was not correctly recognizing the projection of the patient's infantile object relation. He criticized that the in-treatment acting-out of Searles, the therapist, did not enhance the patient's ego.

(4) Summary

Based on the basic perspective on schizophrenia in classical psychoanalysis starting with S. Freud, I presented a historical overview of studies that has developed mainly in the United States to date, except for K. Abraham. This is one of the two major trends in schizophrenia studies and has also had a major impact on Japanese psychoanalysts. The other major trend is the Kleinian school in the United Kingdom.

There are also studies of the independent school by psychoanalysts including Winnicott, and M. Little, but there are not many studies compared to those of the Kleinian school. They consider that the psychotic state is in the period of holding. They think that verbal intervention is meaningless, and maintenance of the therapeutic structure and the therapist's attitude that ensures absolute care to fulfil omnipotent needs are important.

6. M. Klein's Studies on Schizophrenia

(1) Psychoanalysis for children

From 1920 to 1934, M. Klein conducted psychoanalysis for severely ill children aged 2 to 3 years. In the world of psychoanalysis at that time, S. Freud and other analysts considered that such young children were in the pre-Oedipus stage and were incapable of developing transferences because they did not have an inner world, and were not subject to psychoanalytic therapy. The emphasis was on education and guidance for parents.

In 1920, M. Klein began to conduct play therapy including psychoanalysis for children in Budapest, Hungary, under S. Ferenczi. Ferenczi had had a deep interest in infant psychology and had continued research, and was the first to recommend M. Klein to conduct psychoanalysis for children. In 1921, M. Klein moved to Berlin and began to study psychoanalysis for children under K. Abraham. Abraham had provided psychoanalytic treatment for manic-depressive illness in inpatients, especially adults, and had proposed an infantile early object relational pathological theory of manic-depressive illness based on the libido theory of the oral and anal stages. He, too, advised M. Klein to promote psychoanalytic therapy for very young patients aged 2 to 3 years. He also had a great influence on the development of M. Klein's theory and techniques.

M. Klein conducted play therapy to such young children, and found that their play and actions were comparable to adult verbal free associations. She also discovered that such young children already had an inner world, an ability to develop transferences, and had a superego and Oedipus complex. Klein found that the world of transferences developed by such young children was a world filled with sadism and persecutory anxiety.

In other words, the baby's first object is the mother's breast. The baby idealizes the breast that gives satisfaction and introjects it into the self. On the other hand, the baby violently attacks the breast that gives frustration, and projects its own destructiveness. The baby is then frightened of retaliation and is terrified of persecutory anxiety. The baby does not recognize that the good breast and the bad breast belong to the same person (splitting) and lives in a world of part object relations.

From that time, M. Klein began to consider that the predispositions of adult schizophrenia were attributable to the unconscious continuance of such extremely early developmental conflicts. Additionally, M. Klein later considered that a disorder of the symbol formation process, which was observed in the case of Dick who had autistic symptoms, formed predispositions of schizophrenia.

(2) "Paranoid-schizoid position" and "depressive position"

a Depressive position

In the 1930s, M. Klein applied the knowledge she gained from child psychoanalysis to the treatment of adult manic-depressive illness and made many discoveries. In 1935, she conceptualized the pathological object relation of manic-depressive illness as a "depressive position". She states that the depressive position would be seen in babies around the age of six months and would gradually be completed by the age of two. She paid particular attention to the conflicts in the early stages of the "depressive position". It is characterized by a strong ambivalence to the object. Babies have strong affection for good internal objects and intense hatred for bad internal objects. They experience intense conflict (a whole object relation) by becoming aware that these objects are two aspects of the same object. The conflict includes fear of losing an object, intense guilt, and passion for the object. Relatively primitive defence mechanisms such as projection and introjection are active there. At this time, the super-ego already exists and early Oedipus complex begins. As for pathologies such as manic-depressive illness, it is assumed that there lies a problem of fixation to a relatively early stage in the depressive position. In addition, M. Klein focused on manic defence. It is a way for the patient to avoid depressive anxiety by denying the painful reality, demeaning the object, and negating that he/she is dependent on the object.

b Paranoid-schizoid position

In 1946, M. Klein advocated the concept of the "paranoid-schizoid position" based on psychoanalytic cases of schizophrenia. At that time, M. Klein had the opportunity to listen to many cases of psychoanalytic treatment for schizophrenia through supervision from analysts including H.

Rosenfeld. Based on them, she tried clarifying the fixation point of schizophrenia. The "paranoid-schizoid position" is the disposition of babies from birth to six-months of age where the peak is around 3 months of age. It is a world that has much in common with the world filled with persecutory anxiety and sadism which were observed in children's play therapy. Babies live in a world of part object relations. They cannot recognize the mother's body as a whole, and cannot capture that the mother's breasts, face, hands and other parts of the body belong to the same person. In addition, in terms of time, babies cannot recognize that the breast and the face that are giving them satisfaction now are the same as the ones that gave them frustration a while ago. The first important object for the babies is the mother's breast. Babies project the "live instincts" onto the satisfying breast to create an ideal "good object" and direct strong affection to it. Babies then introject that good object into their selves and make it the core of their selves. On the other hand, when the breast is dissatisfying when babies are hungry, they project the "death instinct", that is, aggression, on the object breast to form a "bad object". Babies develop intense hatred and try to foreclose the bad object to the outside world to keep it away as much as possible. Babies also project their aggression onto the object and possess a "persecutory anxiety" that they would be attacked and retaliated by the object and annihilate. The primitive defence mechanisms seen at that time include splitting, introjection, projection, projective identification, denial, and omnipotence.

When the baby is healthy, the good object relations surpass the bad object relations and are integrated into the depressive position to further develop. However, in the opposite case, the world of psychotic conflict will continue unconsciously in a split-off state without being integrated, and will form predispositions for subsequent schizophrenia.

M. Klein heightened the momentum for psychoanalytic treatment for schizophrenia among her colleagues by theorizing such internal object relations in schizophrenia, that is, by clarifying the origin of the transferences.

7. Development of studies on schizophrenia by M. Klein's disciples

From the time M. Klein proposed her innovative concept of "paranoid-schizoid position", her disciples began to actively study analytical treatment for schizophrenia. The representative researchers are H. Rosenfeld, H. Segal, and W. Bion. In particular, the 1950s was the time when clinical studies on schizophrenia were conducted most energetically, and many innovative discoveries were made. Those studies confirmed that the "paranoid-schizoid position" proposed by M. Klein was the fixation point in schizophrenia, and the world of the primitive object relation was reproduced through "psychotic transferences" to the therapist. It is a part object relation, and a world where intense aggression and persecutory anxiety intertwine, and primitive defence mechanisms such as splitting, projection, introjection, omnipotence, denial, and furthermore, projective identification are active. The analysts showed that it was possible and technically important to deal with such patients by interpreting transferences without modifying the psychoanalytic techniques. In fact, they adhered to the basic setting of psychoanalysis, that is a therapeutic structure of 50 minutes, 5 to 6 times a week, and centred on transference interpretations avoiding modified techniques such as support and assurance as much as possible.

(1) H. Rosenfeld — First successful case of psychoanalysis for schizophrenia

a Clinical techniques and theory

In 1947, H. Rosenfeld (1909-1986) reported a psychoanalytic treatment case of schizophrenia with depersonalization. In the treatment, he adhered to the psychoanalytic setting and used techniques that retained transference interpretations. However, as in children's play therapy, he did not instruct the schizophrenic patient to lie down on the couch or give free associations. H. Rosenfeld's description of the treatment course is extremely detailed and varied. He focused mainly on the patient's fragmented linguistic expressions, actions and behaviours to understand the inner world of the patient who could hardly give out linguistic expressions and tried to unravel the patient's world of inner phantasies. He states that the treatment for schizophrenia is more similar to children's play therapy than the treatment for adult neurosis, because it is more necessary to focus on the expressions by actions and behaviours than the means of verbal expression. In other words, in addition to the above-mentioned characteristics, the treatment motives of schizophrenic patients are often ambiguous, and external assistance including hospitalization and support from family members and social workers is often required.

Rosenfeld also considered that various "psychotic transferences" would develop if the therapist focused on interpreting transferences without aiming to develop positive transferences by providing support or assurance.

However, he considered that just understanding the pathology of schizophrenia should be the central goal and it was too early to draw a conclusion about the therapeutic effect on schizophrenia. This was because although there are cases where treatment for schizophrenia can be prominently successful in certain patients, in many cases, there are no other choices but to discontinue therapy because extremely difficult resistances occur or external reality interrupts.

Nevertheless, he continued to have enthusiasm for analytical research on schizophrenia until he passed away in 1986. He accumulated successful therapeutic experiences in many patients with schizophrenia and continued to published important papers.

In the analysis record of a super-ego conflict in an acute schizophrenic patient, which he wrote in 1952, here too, he described the patient's activity and transferences of projective identification in great details, and recorded how much he was trying to understand the subtle patient communications. He stated that such a patient's super-ego was primitive, was very sensitive to guilt, and would immediately be projected to the outside world. Rosenfeld elucidated there was a tendency that the patient would feel persecutory guilt as if the outside world was reproaching him/her. Furthermore, Rosenfeld recorded in minute details of the patient fearing persecutory anxiety since the destructiveness of the patient was projected to the outside world, violently attacking such an object, and later suffering from guilt. Rosenfeld depicted the splitting of the ego and the collapse of the ego, and the patient being terrified of the destruction of the outside world and the destruction of the self's inner world. Patients cannot tolerate guilt and project the internal object, that is the part of the self that had the painful experience caused by the super-ego, to the object and end up losing their self and becoming emotionless.

As shown in his previous paper, an astonishing understanding of such a psychotic world of an acute patient is exhibited based on subtle actions, behaviours, and fragmentary verbal expressions shown at the therapeutic site.

In addition, Rosenfeld said that understanding the subtle communication of schizophrenic patients required the therapists to use their intuition, and to do this, the therapist needs to agilely use his/her counter-transferences. Attention is focused on the normal function of counter-transference here, and he clarified the function of counter-transference in understanding communication of the patient's unconsciousness.

b Studies on the confusional state

H. Rosenfeld focused on the point that during psychoanalytic treatment, patients with chronic schizophrenia would fall into a confusional state. At such times, the patients cannot distinguish sexual drives from aggressive drives, and good objects from bad objects. Drives, objects, and the ego are in a confusional state. Rosenfeld gave an example of a patient who dreamt that one part of his ego ate up another part of his ego, and considered that it was one of the moves of the confusional state.

He also pointed out that there were two ways for the confusional state to resolve. In one way, the ego regains the ability to distinguish things and begins to develop. In the other way, the pathological splitting functions and anxiety disappears. However, the patient's condition becomes worse, and he/she cannot distinguish normally and his/her development stops. Rosenfeld considered that this was a case when the sexual drive succumbed to the aggressive drive and the repair function did not work anymore.

c Studies on narcissistic organization

From the mid-1960s, H. Rosenfeld paid attention to the existence of a narcissistic defence organization in patients characterized by *hikikomori*. He said that such a defence organization could be seen in a wide range of patients, from patients with relatively mild schizoid personalities who are socially adapted to patients with schizophrenia who are in an omnipotent delusional hallucinatory state. He called this defence organization as narcissistic organization and clarified its characteristics. That is, the narcissistic organization is a defence organization where the patient tries not to recognize that he/she is afraid to depend on the object and lose it by overestimating his/her self and despising the object, in order to avoid the painful experience regarding separation from the object. In malignant cases, the part of the self that attacks the object is idealized, and the self is dominated by such a part. In such a state, the self refuses to have a relationship with the object by destructively attacking the part of the self that seeks and depends on the object, and locks itself up in an omnipotent world of narcissism. H. Rosenfeld explained the mechanism of autism in schizophrenia with the concept of such latter destructive narcissistic organization. Of course, it can be seen in other severe personality-disorders in greater or lesser degrees.

d On projective identification

In 1971, Rosenfeld re-emphasized the importance of the mechanism of projective identification in schizophrenic patients and briefly summarized its characteristics. He also referred to studies by W. Bion and H. Segal. First, among the projective identifications found in psychotic patients, there is a healthy and realistic projective identification which is the same projective identification used for normal non-verbal communication between the baby and the mother. Secondly, there is one that is used to remove the part which the self does not desire and to eliminate the psychic reality. Thirdly, there is one used to control the therapist's body and mind, which is very commonly seen in the transferences of psychotic patients. This is based on an extremely early object relation of babies. Fourthly, there is one that is used to deal with primitive aggression, especially envy. Fifthly, there is one that is used by the patient to be confident that he/she is completely living parasitically in the therapist. The second to the fifth projective identifications are pathological projective identification.

e Summary

As described above, H. Rosenfeld's study on schizophrenia was based on his extremely energetic and precise clinical observations and understandings. He brilliantly described that M. Klein's phenomenon of the "paranoid-schizoid position" was lively revived in psychotic transferences. He himself took pride in creating this concept together with Klein, and did not present much more new concepts as Bion did. However, it can be said that Rosenfeld enriched the content of the concept of psychotic transferences, which is a manifestation of the paranoid-schizoid position, and his clinical descriptions are more affluent than those of H. Segal and W. Bion. It was his original idea that narcissistic organizations had something in common with narcissism seen in psychosis and were also related to negative therapeutic responses, thus he made a great contribution to the understanding of treatment for schizophrenia.

(2) H. Segal — Study of symbolization and state of depression in schizophrenia

a Clinical situations

H. Segal (1918–2011) made great efforts to introduce M. Klein's works, and her introductory book is very famous. She also made a significant contribution to the studies on schizophrenia.

She has reported in great detail a successful case of a full-scale psychoanalytic treatment for an in-hospital schizophrenic patient. She too confirmed that the disposition of what M. Klein noted, that is the "paranoid-schizoid position", would appear in transferences. H. Segal especially paid attention to the fact that the patient's symbolic function was impaired and the symbol itself was experienced as the same as concrete things. She considered that such patients were not able to develop their thoughts. Later on, she came to give consideration on this symbolic function with the concept of "symbolic equation". As she additionally mentioned later, H. Segal did not discuss much on her perspective on projective identification and fragmentation of the self.

b Symbolic equation

H. Segal focused on the impaired symbolic process of schizophrenic patients and addressed the characteristics. She gave a consideration on the process of symbol formation based on M. Klein's developmental theory of the "paranoid-schizoid position" and the "depressive position". She grasped the concept of symbolism broadly as an expression in place of an object, and discussed the problem of symbols in patients with schizophrenia, which differed in quality from what was commonly seen. Patients with schizophrenia have an inner world of the "paranoid-schizoid position". For example, a schizophrenic patient could not play the guitar because he regarded that playing the guitar in public was the same thing as masturbating in public. This is different from a neurotic patient admitting in associations that playing the guitar represented masturbation for him. In the latter case, the patient has an ability to distinguish between symbols and what is symbolized.

H. Segal named the primitive symbolic function, which is seen in the former case, as a "symbolic equivalent" and tried to express the characteristics. It is related to the "paranoid-schizoid position", a state in which the self, the object and the symbol are not clearly distinguished because of pathological projective identification. There, what is symbolized and the symbol are treated as equivalent concrete objects. It is related to the concrete thinking which is characteristic of schizophrenic patients. They often have impaired abstract thinking because this symbolic function remains in a primitive state.

According to H. Segal, symbols are formed for the ego to deal with the anxiety that arose in the relationship with the object. In addition, symbol formation begins very early when the object relations begin, but its properties change as the object relations change. H. Segal thought that the symbolic process was a good reflection of the state of ego and object relations. Therefore, when the relation with the object is impaired, the symbol formation is also impaired. In particular, when the distinction between the ego and the object is impaired, the distinction between the symbol and the symbolized object is impaired, and this brings about concrete thinking characteristic in schizophrenic patients.

When we reach the "depressive position", the symbolic function is completed. It is a whole object relation, and there is a clear distinction between ego, object and symbol. Symbolic equations and symbols are clearly distinguished there. Symbols are needed to replace aggression against the object and they reduce guilt and the fear of object loss. When we experience object loss, the ability to regenerate that object in the inner world gives the power to use symbols freely. Then, symbols become representations of the object.

Symbols are the protagonists of communication, and all communications are conducted by symbols. When a schizophrenic mechanism works, the symbolic function does not work well. For example, words, whether those of the patient or the therapist, are perceived as objects or actions and are not used aptly in communication. Symbols are also important for internal communication, and when the symbolic function is impaired, internal communication is impaired. We individuals can only have contact with ourselves when we have a free symbolic function. Treating schizophrenic patients is difficult not only because it is difficult to communicate with them, but also because the patients cannot communicate with their own inner world.

Communicating with ourselves through this symbolic function becomes the basis of verbal thinking. Although not all internal communications are conducted through verbal thinking, all verbal thinking is internal communication using a symbol called language.

c Studies on depression in schizophrenia

H. Segal discussed depression that appeared in the course of psychoanalytic treatment for patients with schizophrenia. As always, she gave a minute detailed clinical description of how the patient transitioned and reversed the "paranoid-schizoid position", where the schizoid mechanism is active, to the "depressive position" world. When persecutory anxiety and schizoid defences are delt with in treatment, the ego and the object come to integrate, and the patient's reality-testing ability improves. This leads the patient to possess depressed feelings and guilt and feel the need for reparation. Such emotions become difficult for the patient to tolerate, and the patient immediately projects and splits-off the depressive part of self to the object, that is, the therapist, by the mechanism of projective identification. Then the therapist will have the depressive experience. The patient's sane part is removed, and a persecutory world arises again. What is therapeutically important is to clarify this process in transferences.

(3) W. Bion — The genetic construction of the psychotic personality theory

a Study situation

W. Bion (1897-1979) had similar clinical experiences with those in the world of abundant clinical observation and description of analysts including H. Rosenfeld and H. Segal as described above. He then theoretically summarized those observations from a new perspective and succeeded in unravelling the complex world of psychosis. The above two analysts did not use many other concepts except for M. Klein's "paranoid-schizoid position" and tried to understand the world of psychotic transferences within that framework. In contrary, Bion used his own unique concept to elucidate the world of schizophrenia to theorize the more detailed observations. W. Bion appeared in the felid of psychoanalysis a little later and was not much involved in the timing when the concepts of the positions were formed, so it seems that he was active in forming a new concept. In a sense, it can be said that W. Bion was the analyst who made the most unique contribution among the three.

b "Psychotic personality" and "non-psychotic personality"

Through his experience treating patients with schizophrenia, W. Bion discovered that a psychotic personality and a non-psychotic personality (i.e., neurotic or normal personality) existed simultaneously in such patients. This finding was based on Freud's perspective. Bion found that when the patients' psychotic symptoms were in the foreground, the psychotic personality was in the forefront and the non-psychotic personality was latent in the background. Conversely, in patients with severe neurosis and borderline cases, the non-psychotic personality part is in the foreground and a psychotic personality exists in the background. Bion considered that those patients often undergo a mental breakdown because that psychotic personality would activate.

According to Bion, this psychotic part develops to cope with the situation where the baby cannot tolerate the anxiety of annihilation associated with very early frustration. Babies are, for example, exposed to intense frustration when breasts to feed them do not appear immediately when they are hungry. When they cannot tolerate the painful reality, they try to deal with it by destroying their ego function that recognizes that reality. In other words, they try to avoid experiencing such a painful reality by destroying parts of their ego including sense impression, thoughts, language function, and symbolic function.

It is an energized activity of excessive schizoid mechanism and pathological projective identification. The ego fragments parts of the ego such as sense impressions, thoughts, and words (excessive splitting) and projects them into the outside world to form "bizarre objects". They contain a fragment of the self, but are experienced as things. Since bizarre objects include self-aggression, they become the basis of persecutory delusions. The ego re-introjects them and tries to use them in the self's thoughts, but when they return through the sensory organs, they become hallucinatory experiences.

As described above, when such a psychotic personality begins to be active, the patient is clinically in a state of psychotic transference. When patients encounter abandonment experiences, intense anger, depressive experiences, and painful experiences and cannot deal with them well, the psychotic personality often activates. This is a state which M. Klein theorized as the "paranoid-schizoid position". W. Bion succeeded in explaining it in a genetic and formative manner, and developmentally clarified why symbolic function, thought, and language function are impaired in a psychotic sate.

c Container/contained relationship and projective identification

As mentioned above, W. Bion stated that pathological projective identification played a major role in the formation and activity of a psychotic personality. On the other hand, he focused on healthy projective identification. It is basically important for communication between the baby and the mother. The baby projects anxiety and conflict that he/she cannot deal with on to his/her mother. The mother who receives them reads the meaning by "reverie", makes it into something that the baby can deal with, and returns it to the baby. The baby will now experience it as something he/she can accept, introjects it as his/her self's experience (introjective identification), and comes to be able to use it as an ingredient for thoughts, dreams, and representations. W. Bion called this relationship between the baby and the mother a container-contained relationship, and elucidated that the mother's function played a major role for a healthy mental development. The communication between the mother and the baby is based on a healthy projective identification there. This healthy projective identification also plays an important role as functions in adults such as sympathizing, empathizing, and intuitive understanding, and is the basis for the world of emotional interaction.

Furthermore, in clinical practice, projective identification also contributes to the understanding of counter-transferences. Counter-transference includes healthy counter-transference such as emotions and thoughts that arise in the therapist due to the patient's communication. The healthy counter-transference is understood by exchanging projective identifications between the therapist and the patient. It is a subtle communication that does not involve symbolic functions such as language. How this information can be used therapeutically is an important issue in the treatment for psychotic patients and other serious patients.

The other counter-transference arises from the therapist's personal unresolved conflicts, as mentioned by S. Freud which should be resolved by training analysis and self-analysis.

d Studies on thoughts

W. Bion focused on thought disorders in schizophrenia and made a developmental consideration. Here, W. Bion put forward a hypothesis that, babies are born dispositionally with a "preconception" of, for example, the breast and when what the babies want are actually given to them and their desire is realized (realization), a "conception" occurs and when this is repeated, it becomes a "concept". On the premise of that hypothesis, Bion made a developmental consideration on the formation of thoughts. If the baby is not given his/her desired breast, "conception" of the "absent breast" occurs. W. Bion named this case of unrealized "conception" accompanying frustration as "thought". Thoughts inevitably require "thinking" since the meanings are linked.

However, in order for this thought to be formed, the baby must be able to withstand the frustration of the absence of the breast. W. Bion considered that this tolerance is also greatly influenced by predisposing factors. If the baby's tolerance is sufficient, the experience is conceptualized and the baby can learn from it. If the baby is less tolerant of frustration and the baby cannot stand the absence of the breast, the preconceptions and negative thoughts about the experience become bad objects, and they are fragmented, shattered and projected to the outside world and experienced as "a thing". As a result, all thoughts become indistinguishable from internal bad objects and are subject to splitting. This will form "bizarre objects" and the world of psychotic personality will evolve. As a result, thoughts are impaired, and this brings about a major obstacle to communication. In such cases, patients develop omnipotent thoughts and omnipotence instead of conception and become unable to distinguish truth from falsity.

Moreover, not only the baby's predisposition problems, but also the mother's quality of a balanced understanding and cooperation with the baby influences the formation of thoughts from the mother's environment. In other words, if the baby projects what he/she wants to remove onto the mother's breast, and the mother properly understands and deals with it and returns it to the baby in an alleviated manner, the baby can tolerate the experience and develop his/her thoughts by introjectively identifying the experience as a part of his/her self. This is the above-mentioned mother's function of reverie and container. W. Bion called the function of changing the sensory data so that the baby can use the experience for dream thought with the cooperation and understanding of the mother, that is, the function of changing the data into "alpha elements", as the "alpha function". If this mother's function does not work well, the baby will not be able to use the sense impressions for mental development, and will form "beta elements" or "bizarre objects".

As described above, W. Bion considered that the predispositions for schizophrenia were influenced by both the baby's constitutional genetic factors and the mother's reverie function and container function.

From the latter half of the 1960s, W. Bion developed ontological semiotics represented by grids, but this paper will omit this subject.

(4) J. Steiner — Studies on pathological organization

J. Steiner was influenced by H. Rosenfeld's narcissistic organization and compiled a more comprehensive personality theory. He called it a pathological organization. This theory contributed significantly to the understanding of the world of pathology, especially in psychotic patients and severe borderline cases. It provides a guideline to understand and deal with patients who show difficult-to-treat negative therapeutic responses.

a Pathological organization as a third position This pathological organization is a third position which is different from the healthy paranoid-schizoid position and depressive position. It functions also as a kind of a place for "retreating" and is also a nest for pathological object relations. It shows a strong resistance against the development of healthy positions and is in a unique equilibrium state. It also acts as a defence organization that strongly resists treatment and plays a major role in the formation of a pathological personality.

b Diversity of pathological organization

Clinically, the pathological organizations have a broad spectrum ranging from obsessive, manic-depressive, perverted, to psychotic conditions. Depending on the condition, the state of the internal pathological organizations shows how object relations are; they vary from neurotic, perverted, manic-depressive, to psychotic object relations. Pathological organizations are the source of pathological object relations and, developmentally, are the worlds of pathological object relations which have gradually been formed in the self from the patients' infancy through the repetition of projective identification and introjective identification of destructive and atrocious object relations with the objects. In the case of psychotic pathological organizations, persecutory anxiety is prominent due to fragmentation of the ego and the object and excessive projective identification. Cognitive impairment, language function impairment, and thought function disorder are seen, and also the patients are in a state of delusional hallucination. Steiner, following Bion, associated schizophrenia with the presence of a psychotic personality and concluded that it was one of the spectrums of all personality disorders.

Steiner described the main common characteristics of these pathological organizations as follows: (1) They strongly resist change and are in an equilibrium state. (2) Projective identification and a pathological defence mechanism of splitting are active. Therefore, persecutory anxiety and abandonment anxiety are prominent. (3) They differ from the two healthy positions and are pathological. (4) The internal object relations are perverted and addictive. (5) They are narcissistic and their destructiveness is often idealized. In contrast to the tendency of other healthy selves which recognize the value of the therapist, depend on him/her and try to change developmentally, pathological organizations destructively deal with and control the therapist, and strongly resist change.

In the case of psychotic personality, there is a corresponding pathological organization in the background, and strong persecutory anxiety as well as impaired ego boundaries and impaired thoughts and language function become apparent due to fragmentation and excessive projective identification.

c Development of the position theory

J. Steiner divided M. Klein's developmental stages of the positions into four stages in order to further sort out the content of these pathological organizations in pathological personalities: (1) Early paranoid-schizoid position (characterized by fragmentation and annihilation anxiety), (2) Late paranoid-schizoid position (characterized by splitting and persecutory anxiety), (3) Early depressive position (characterized by abandonment fear and persecutory guilt), (4) Late depressive position (characterized by mourning work and mourning). Steiner thought that the pathological condition such as psychosis, manic depression, perversion, borderline case, or neurosis, differed depending on the timing when the pathological organization was formed in the developmental line. When the pathological organization is psychotic, he considered that the pathological object relation was organized during the early paranoid-schizoid position or the late paranoid-schizoid position.

Therapeutically, the object relations of such pathological organizations are often transferred and acted out during treatment. It is important for the therapist to carefully ascertain how much a destructive relation it is in with the developmental process of the healthy positions. It is also essential for the therapist to understand how the transferences of the internal object relations in pathological organizations are occurring. They need to be handled with interpretation. In the case of psychotic pathological organizations, psychotic transferences develop, so it becomes therapeutically important to carefully interpret the anxiety and primitive defence activities.

(5) Summary

I have summarized the Kleinian studies on schizophrenia in line with the historical trend. They have treated many schizophrenic patients with techniques that focus on the interpretation of psychotic transferences, without changing the psychoanalytic techniques as much as possible. Some of the patients they reported in detail exhibited significant improvement, which indicated that psychoanalysis was effective for some patients. However, as H. Rosenfeld clearly stated, not all patients with schizophrenia can be treated successfully. Even if their pathology seems to be understandable, treatment may be interrupted due to severe resistance in some cases. In that sense, psychoanalytic treatment for schizophrenia is still at the stage of research. Nevertheless, what has been elucidated in the treatments has made a great contribution to the understanding of patients with other severe personality disorders. Also, in my experience, there are patients with psychotic episodes and apparent psychotic personality who therapeutically fall into a psychotic breakdown or present psychotic transferences but therapeutically respond extremely well to a psychoanalytic approach. The future challenge is to accumulate clinical experiences of analytical treatment for schizophrenia and find out what kind of patients are suitable for psychoanalysis and its criteria.

8. Diagnosis and therapeutic techniques for psychogenic schizophrenia (psychotic personality)

(1) Differentiation of psychogenic schizophrenia

Not all patients diagnosed as schizophrenia are subject to psychoanalytic therapy. Practically, we take sufficient time for diagnostic interviews (usually four 45-to-50-minute sessions) to obtain multifaceted information regarding the patient and diagnose psychogenic schizophrenia, that is, psychotic personality. Sometimes, we refer to psychological tests and drawing tests. The general characteristics are as follows: (1) The patient has a conflictual unique episode in his/her life history. (2) Many of the parent images are relatively conflicting, for example they conducted violent and verbal attacks, and many of the parents themselves have experiences of deprivation. (3) A specific counter-transference occurs where the therapist feels that psychotherapy may be better for the patient. (4) When the therapist recommends psychotherapy to the patient at that time, the patient accepts it.

In general, there are patients who have a strong biophysiological tendency in schizophrenic patients, which is called the core group. However, among the patients called the peripheral group, there are the above-mentioned psychogenic patients (psychotic personality) and there is a group that can be improved by a psychoanalytic approach.

(2) Therapeutic structure

The therapeutic structure for psychotic personality is no different from that in general psychoanalytic therapy. An approach centring on transference interpretations is taken without modifying the basic techniques. The therapist takes an appropriate neutral attitude and works to capture subtle communication activities in the patient's psychotic expressions. Even though patients often develop psychotic breakdowns or psychotic transferences, it becomes an important therapeutic act to understand the subtle communication based on the patient's primitive anxiety and interpret it to the patient. In that case, it is also extremely essential to understand the patient's non-verbal communication through counter-transferences.

9. Conclusion

I have given an overview of the history of psychoanalytic treatment for and pathology of schizophrenia. I also introduced the trend of psychoanalytic treatment for psychosis, which developed mainly in the United States by Federn, Sulliven, From-Reichman, Searles and other analysts. They were influenced by S. Freud's therapeutic nihilism, and tried to succeed S. Freud's basic idea. Next, I introduced another huge trend, the Kleinian studies which arose from Abraham and was developed by analysts such as Klein, Rosenfeld, Segal, Bion and Steiner. They are a group that has argued that it is important to therapeutically interpret psychotic transferences without changing the basic psychoanalytic setting. In order to do so, I stated that psychogenic schizophrenia and psychotic personality should be differentiated by assessment and targeted for psychoanalytic therapy. In any case, adopting a therapeutic approach to the world of psychosis with psychoanalysis poses many difficulties and unknown worlds, and many of them are still in the research stage. However, many things have been elucidated by the tireless efforts of our predecessors, and it is gradually becoming possible to understand the world of psychosis.

References

(1) Abraham, Karl. 1979. *Selected Papers on Psychoanalysis*. London: Hogarth Press.

(2) Bion, Wilfred Ruprecht. 1957. "Differentiation of the Psychotic from the Non-Psychotic Personalities". *International Journal of Psychoanalysis*, Vol. 38 (3-4): 266-275.

(3) Bion, Wilfred Ruprecht. 1962. "A Theory of Thinking". *International Journal of Psychoanalysis*, Vol. 43: 306-310.

(4) Bion, Wilfred Ruprecht. 1967. *Second Thoughts*. London: Heineman.

(5) Bion, Wilfred Ruprecht. 1977. *Seven Servants.* New York: Jason Aronson.

(6) Federn, Paul. 1953. *Ego Psychology and the Psychoses*. New York: Basic Books.

(7) Freud, Sigmund. 1907. "Delusions and Dreams in Jensen's "Gradiva"". In *Standard Edition*, Vol. 9: 1-95. London: Hogard Press.
(8) Freud, Sigmund. 1911a. "Formulation on the Two Principles of Mental Functioning". In *Standard Edition*, Vol. 12: 215-226. London: Hogard Press.
(9) Freud, Sigmund. 1911b. "Psycho Analytic Notes on an Autobiographic Account of a Case of Paranoia (Dementia Paranoides)". In *Standard Edition*, Vol. 12: 3-82. London: Hogard Press.
(10) Freud, Sigmund. 1914. "On narcissism: An introduction". In *Standard Edition*, Vol. 12: 215-226. London: Hogard Press.
(11) From-Reichman, Frieda. 1959. *Psychoanalysis and Psychotherapy: Selected papers of Frieda Fromm-Reichmann*. Chicago: The University of Chicago Press.
(12) Kinugasa, Takayuki. 1991. "Psychopathology of Schizophrenia; in view of Bion". *The Japanese Journal of Psycho-analysis*, Vol. 35, No. 3: 224-235 (in Japanese)
(13) Kinugasa, Takayuki. 1992. "On Schizophrenia Under the Kleinian View". *Imago*, Vol. 3, No. 11. Tokyo: Seidosha (in Japanese)
(14) Kinugasa, Takayuki. 1998. "On the Formation of the Body Images in Psychosis — In Kleinian Thoughts —". *The Japanese Journal of Psycho-analysis*, Vol. 42, No. 2: 129-136 (in Japanese) (Chapter 3 of this book (in English))
(15) Kinugasa, Takayuki. 2002. "Psychoanalysis of Schizophrenia". *Schizophrenia Frontier*, Vol. 3, No. 2, 12-17 (in Japanese)
(16) Klein, Melanie. 1930. "The Importance of Symbol-Formation in the Development of the Ego". In *The Writings of Melanie Klein*, Vol. 1. London: Hogarth Press.
(17) Klein, Melanie. 1932/1975. "Psychoanalysis of Children". In *The Writings of Melanie Klein*, Vol. 2. London: Hogarth Press.
(18) Klein, Melanie. 1935/1975. "A Contribution to the Psychogenesis of Manic-Depressive States". In *The Writings of Melanie Klein*, Vol. 1. London: Hogarth Press.
(19) Klein, Melanie. 1946/1975. "Notes on Some Schizoid Mechanisms". In *The Writings of Melanie Klein*, Vol. 3, 1-24. London: Hogarth Press.
(20) Okonogi, Keigo. 1985a. *Clinical Challenges of Psychoanalysis*. Tokyo: Kongo-shuppan (in Japanese)
(21) Okonogi, Keigo. 1985b. Tokyo: *The Origin and Development of Psychoanalysis*. Koubundou Publisher (in Japanese)

(22) Okonogi, Keigo. 1992. "Schizophrenia Seen from Psychoanalysis". *Imago*, Vol. 3, No. 11. Tokyo: Seidosha (in Japanese)
(23) Rosenfeld, Herbert. 1947/1965. "Analysis of a Schizophrenic State with Depersonalization". In *Psychotic States*, 13-33. London: Hogarth Press.
(24) Rosenfeld, Herbert. 1950. "Notes on the Psychopathology of Confusional States in Chronic Schizophrenia". In *Psychotic States*. London: Hogarth Press.
(25) Rosenfeld, Herbert. 1952/1985. "Notes on the Psycho-Analysis of the Superego Conflict in an Acute Schizophrenic Patient". In *Psychotic States*. London: Karnac Books.
(26) Rosenfeld, Herbert. 1964/1965. "On the Psychopathology of Narcissism: A Clinical Approach". In *Psychotic States*. London: Hogarth Press.
(27) Rosenfeld, Herbert. 1965. *Psychotic States*. London: Hogarth Press.
(28) Rosenfeld, Herbert. 1969. "On the Treatment of Psychotic States by Psychoanalysis: An Historical Approach". *International Journal of Psychoanalysis*, Vol. 50: 615-631.
(29) Rosenfeld, Herbert. 1971/1988. "Contribution to the Psychopathology of Psychotic States: The Importance of Projective Identification in the Ego Structure and the Object Relations of the Psychotic Patient". In *Melanie Klein Today*, Vol. 1. London: Routledge.
(30) Rosenfeld, Herbert. 1987. *Impasse and Interpretation*. London: Tavistock Publications.
(31) Searles, Harold. 1963. *Collected Papers on Schizophrenia and Related Subjects*. London: Hogarth Press.
(32) Segal, Hanna. 1950. "Some Aspects of the Analysis of a Schizophrenic". *International Journal of Psychoanalysis*, Vol. 31: 268-278.
(33) Segal, Hanna. 1957/1981. "Notes on Symbol Formation". *International Journal of Psychoanalysis*, Vol. 38: 391-397. Also, in *The Work of Hanna Segal*. New York: Jason Aronson.
(34) Segal, Hanna. 1981. *The Work of Hanna Segal*. New York: Jason Aronson
(35) Spillius, Elizabeth Bott. 1988: *Melanie Klein Today*, Vol. 1. London: Routledge.
(36) Steiner, John. 1991. "A Psychotic Organization of the Personality". *International Journal of Psychoanalysis*, Vol. 72: 201-207.
(37) Steiner, John. 1993. *Psychic Retreats*. London: Routledge.
(38) Sullivan, Harry. 1962. *Schizophrenia as a Human Process*. New York: Norton & Company.

[2004. *The Japanese Journal of Psycho-analysis*, Vol. 48, No. 1.]

ON THEORIES

CHAPTER 8

WHAT ARE CLINICAL FACTS? THE PROCESS FROM RECORDING TO PRESENTING THE CLINICAL PROCESS

1. Introduction

In the process of recording and summarizing what we therapists experience in the treatment of patients and presenting them in clinical papers, a psychic, subjective, and proactive relationship built on the transference-countertransference relationship between the therapist and the patient becomes the basis. By examining what is happening in this process step by step, I would like to consider how we therapists experience clinical facts, and what kind of experiences we go through when organizing them into clinical papers. The consideration on the treatment process is based on the modern Kleinian techniques which the author actually practices.

2. Basic problems of clinical facts

The matter of clinical facts is common to not only the therapists with perspectives of the Kleinian theory and techniques, like the author, but all therapists who practice clinical activities from various perspectives of psychoanalysis. This issue is, in a sense, an issue that includes all the methodologies and theories of psychoanalysis. Therapists become involved in the issue of the specific character of psychoanalytic methodologies, and are confronted by the matter of difference between natural science and human science. It has to do with the matter of how we recognize, understand, and perceive the minds of others, and it is naturally different from the way we recognize non-human objects, that is, the material world. We interact with others on the premise that they have a mind. However, the mind of others is something considered to exist beyond their various expressions perceived by our sight and hearing. It is probably something that is perceived by a healthy projective identification or intuition and empathy based on, in a sense, our "concept of humans". However, we cannot observe the minds of others with certain solidity as existences that act directly on our visual, auditory and tactile senses, as we can observe substances. We perceive the minds of others intuitively, affectively, emotionally, and conceptually in the interactions with others. It is a process which advances in a delicate intricacy of what constantly changes over time and what retains a homogeneity. A healthy person essentially has an ability to distinguish what is inside the human mind from what is outside. However, in a pathological state, this ability does not work well. The way of being of individual existences changes in various ways and something happens which becomes difficult for others to understand. Although this matter steps into the field of philosophy, the specificity of psychoanalysis is that it extends the field of consideration to the ontology of babies and infants, the ontology of unconsciousness, and the ontology of psychic partial unconsciousness.

3. Facts in psychoanalytic clinical practice

It is quite a difficult task to position facts in psychoanalytic clinical practice. In psychoanalysis, therapists try to understand the unconscious world of the patient through free association and in a specific relationship where the therapist is in a state with "free floating attention". It is based on a method of exploring and trying to understand the world which is expressed symbolically through free association, or the unspoken world between the lines. They often are not directly expressed in words, or are expressed by slips of the tongue, faltering of associations, inscrutable dreams, subtle movements and acting-outs. It can be said that we therapists are saddled with something fatal in our clinical activities that the subjects of our attention are things that are not directly spoken or expressed. This is different from the way to capture physical material existences. In fact, the question about what the facts regarding the human mind are seems to be a question that even philosophers have not solved yet. The facts captured in what occurs in the human world differ according to the viewpoints or methods; for example, facts in the press, facts in court, historical facts, sociological facts, and facts of political science are perceived differently. Thus, it is necessary to have a special method and viewpoint in order to address the invisible and unspoken parts of the unconscious human mind as the subject of understanding. The special method and viewpoint are based on Freud's genius idea where the patient lies on a couch and gives free association while the therapist, who sits behind the patient and maintains a state of "free floating attention", listens attentively to the patient's free associations. There exists a mental fact that cannot be approached unless through this special setting. Here, the basic theoretical viewpoints in psychoanalysis including the unconscious theory, mental structure theory, development theory, and dream theory, come into the picture as something indispensable.

4. Knowing the mind through the mind

In any case, when we understand the mind of others, we can only do so through our own mind. This is a process that is quite different from the process of understanding the nature of substances and the movement of celestial bodies. We have various emotions, ideas, and impressions: At times, we think that we have understood the minds of others, at other times, we feel that we cannot be understood easily, or we feel that we somehow cannot like a person. At such times, the question is "What means and methods can we use to treat the minds and selves of others as if they existed there?" This has been investigated by philosophers and psychoanalysts such as Bion, however, after all, it is assumed to be due to the human's intrinsic capacity to perceive the minds of others, that is comprehension and intuition. In actual treatment for patients, although the relationship between the therapist and the patient has a special stance as described above, these humane capacities of comprehension and intuition are the basis, and we therapists further understand the patients by making full use of our emotions, fantasies, imaginations and other capacities. We mobilize them as much as possible to try to understand the unconscious world that lies beyond the patient's associations. It is very difficult to verify whether the therapist's understanding is correct, and it is a world that can only be confirmed by giving the patient interpretations and validating his/her reaction to the given interpretations.

After all, the world of our human relationships evolves around such elusive things. For example, it is true that babies express emotions through various movements and facial expressions, but communication between the mother and baby is established because of the mother's inbuilt intuitive perceiving capability (dream function; Bion). Through this communication, the baby repeatedly has experiences of satisfaction and happiness and experiences of dissatisfaction and pain, and builds a mental world of self and others. It is surprising that humans' mind and relationships are made up of such things, however, within such a foundation, our world of experiences with others progresses, and the world between us and others will build up as a concrete thing. This is a very strange thing when you think about it, but the world of our minds is active in such a vulnerable world of experiences, and in that world, our mental health and our world of pathology evolve.

Since clinical practice of psychoanalysis deals with such worlds, the process of understanding the unconsciousness of the minds of others is a world of trial and error. The patients' unconscious world that we can glimpse in each session is only an extremely small part of that world. By accumulating those parts, their unconscious world gradually makes an appearance just like a jigsaw puzzle. The therapist captures, with certain conviction, the unconscious world active there through the patient's associations, but even if the therapist experiences that he/she has understood it, it will not always be correct. Sometimes, the interpretations are pertinent and sometimes they are wrong. The reason why the therapist can have certain confidence at that point raises a major question. As Freud states, whether the interpretation is correct or not should not be judged by the patient's positive or negative response, but should be judged by what kind of development the subject of free association shows after the interpretation. Therefore, attention should be paid to what kind of world of new meanings the associations and acting-outs seen after the interpretation unconsciously create. This means that it is important to understand how the unconscious world reacts according to interpretations and what the unconscious responses are. This is a completely different method from how common-sense judgment is made in our ordinary conversations.

This is related to Freud's unconscious world, the world of psychic reality. This is an individual subjective and unconscious world. It is different from external facts, and it is often difficult for even the subject to be conscious of everything. Such a world is the object of our therapists' understanding and recognition. As is often said, this is the world of transference and countertransference, which are the most basic viewpoints of treatment, and we come to deal with the world of delicate exchanges and interactions between two subjective and independent minds. There exist many processes that have not yet been clearly identified.

5. The actual process in the therapist-patient relationship

The therapist takes the patient's overall expressions, such as the patient's content of conversation, movements, tone of speaking, slips of the tongue, lateness or absence, and dreams, as a manifestation of the activity of their unconscious phantasy, and considers them as materials for understanding. There, the therapist clearly is carrying out some kind of perception and cognition, and is making a selection. This means that while the therapist is attentively listening to the patient's associations, he/she is already making a selection from the beginning what is meaningful and what is not. Thus, when the therapist keeps a record after the session is over, there are many parts that have not remained in his/her memory. Matters such as why the therapist can intuitively feel that he/she can understand some parts, why he/she feels some parts do not make sense, or why some parts do not remain in his/her memory, are related to many factors of the therapist. It seems to be related to what is conducted when a person goes through many stages in the process of recognizing and understanding another person. Freud considered that the therapist's individual unresolved conflicts create many blind spots at each therapeutic site and have unfavourable effects on his/her initial cognition and the stage of comprehension. He proposed that the therapist him/herself should receive psychoanalytical treatment as much as possible to reduce the unfavourable effects (educational analysis). This is now one of the most important trainings to become a psychoanalyst. However, there are also other factors in the issue when therapists actually select the patient's materials and give meanings to them.

The therapist recognizes the patient's communication and selects the elements. Some remain in the therapist's consciousness and stimulate his/her unconsciousness. At that point, the therapist sorts out the patient's associations and other expressions into meaningful expressions and meaningless expressions, and some of them fall out from his/her memory for some reason. This is a process in which the elements of the patient's expressions are selected according to a certain intention of the therapist. The selected elements are collected to form a certain meaning. Such a process takes place in the activity where the therapist reads between the lines of the patient's associations and tries to draw close the patient's unconscious world. Then, by accumulating them, the therapist constructs, interprets, and forms a concept of a certain meaning. In addition, it is thought that theorization is carried out while the therapist observes the patient's associations, acting-outs, and other various nonverbal expressions on the time axis and accumulates meaningful ones.

6. The therapist's interpretation and its correctness

The therapist selects information and forms a certain meaning while listening to the patient's associations. At that time, the therapist develops a special kind of conviction, which is brought about by the therapist's intuition, but is not clear whether it is correct or not. Therapy is conducted in a special setting of only two people. In a situation where no third person intervenes, the therapist verbalizes the meaning of the unconscious world which he/she composed as an interpretation to the patient, and judges if it is right or wrong. When doing so, the patient gives various reactions; for example, ignores or strongly denies, or attacks or praises it. At this time, the therapist experiences various emotions such as being hurt, being tickled his/her self-esteem, feeling frank joy, being shaken his/her conviction, or losing him/herself. However, as Freud states above, the therapist will judge whether the interpretation is correct not by the patient's affirmation or denial, but by how the patient's association develops thereafter.

For the therapist, the process of dealing with analytical facts takes place in an extremely unique inner world, or a world where dual subjectivity and independence intersect, that is, a world that looks at the relationship between the patient's inner world and the therapist's inner world. It is a world where the therapist discovers a certain meaning in such world. This is different from the world of facts recorded, for example, by tape recorders or video cameras. This is compared to the relationship between manifest dreams and latent dreams. The world that is happening beyond the world recorded on tape records or other devices is the clinical facts for us therapist.

7. Selection of expression elements by the therapist

How does the therapist select what are expressed by the patient's associations and acting-outs? As mentioned above, a selection is first made at the stage when the therapist recognizes the patient's expressions, but a more aggressive selection is executed secondarily, and the world of meanings is created using them as base materials. At that time, the theoretical viewpoints of psychoanalysis are considered to have a great influence. For Kleinians, the main theories are unconscious phantasy, transference, countertransference, paranoid schizoid position, depressive position, primitive defence mechanisms such as splitting and projective identification, early Oedipus complex, and early superego. The theories of psychoanalysis often are the basic perspectives for the complex clinical pictures. They have influence on where the therapist sees the incidences that happen in clinical practice from, and where he/she focuses on. Although there are various concepts in analysis, the clinical concepts mentioned above play particularly important roles, and many of them have descriptive aspects. In Japanese, the word 'theory' possesses an image of natural science which constructs a theory based on rigorous thinking such as mathematical physical theories, however, the concept of theory in psychoanalysis is humane. Many of the psychoanalytic theories give a certain viewpoint to the movements in clinical practice and half of them have descriptive implications. In the case of Kleinians, the therapeutic structure complies with free association conducted in the lying-down method, and although there are many common points with other schools, the basic viewpoint will be decided by the theoretical concept focusing on the above-mentioned early object relations. When actually selecting elements of free associations and other materials provided by the patient, the elements that are considered to correspond to the developmental theory of the two positions will be selected, and then the world of unconscious phantasy will reveal its concrete meaning. Why such phenomena are therapeutically important has been disputed for a long time among and clinical research have been conducted by psychoanalysts with different theoretical perspectives. There is such clinical importance in psychoanalytic theories and there is such a close relationship with therapeutic techniques.

As described above, it seems that therapists are easily sorting out the elements of the patient's association materials, but in reality, he/she selects them with delicate sensitivity. Not only through theoretical learning, but also through the experience of supervision, experience of educational analysis, and treatment experiences with other patients, a therapeutic mental stance is formed inside the therapist. With that as the axis, the therapist constitutes and verifies the meaning of the patient's world. Then, based on that, the therapist recognizes the patient's world of associations, sifts through what seems to be meaningful, and tries to read the activity of the patient's unconscious world of meaning. It is considered that this meaning-giving is also clearly influenced by the theoretical basic standpoint.

Bion describes this function with the concept of containment. Concretely, the mother (the therapist) introjects what the baby (such part of the patient) projectively identifies to the mother (the therapist), understands the meaning, and returns the meaning to the baby. In this process, what the baby could not introject, that is what the baby could not understand and projectively identified to the mother, is transformed into something meaningful this time by the function of the mother's phantasy, becomes an experience that can be introjected, and will be returned to the baby. They will then be used as materials for the baby's perception, memory, thoughts, and dreams. Similarly, Bion considers the process where the therapist discovers the meaning of the association materials submitted by the patient, transforms it into a meaningful direction, and conveys it to the patient, as an important therapeutic process. He thinks that such an experience world is continuously occurring in the treatment process. When the therapist conveys to the patient meaningful things which the therapist found through the patient's association, and when they resonate with the patient's world, the patient will have an experience of being understood and discovering the meaning together with the therapist. This is significant for mental development and is thought to play a therapeutically important function.

8. Narrative

In this way, clinical facts occur within an extremely subjective and unique relationship between two selves. The therapist's self actively selects and gives meanings to the association materials and other materials of the patient, and scoops up and composes the world of unconscious meanings. Then, as the therapist returns them to the patient in words as interpretations, the therapist tries to create experiences where the patient discovers and shares the world of meanings which he/she could not perceive until then. Clinical work is to repeat the process in which the therapist translates the experiences into words and tells them to the patient, and the patient accordingly gives associations. It is considered that a certain kind of narrative (dialogue) exchanged in this process actually represents clinical facts. The quality of these clinical facts is completely different from that of the facts recorded on tape recorders, as mentioned at the beginning of this paper. It is a narrative created in a world where two independent selves align their souls and share the experience that they are understood by and understand each other in a special kind of collaborative work (although there is a difference in the roles between the therapist and the patient).

Although there are various opinions about this, such a world of narratives has a great influence when describing actual cases. Clinical description will be the work in which the therapist sees what are happening in such an interrelationship from a third person's view and gives meaning to them. It is to introduce a third-person's perspective into the subjective two-party relationship.

9. Conclusion — Publishing papers

We finally come to the stage of clinical description. It seems that there will be even greater restrictions when it comes to publishing. As other authors have stated, various anxiety factors will be added: for example, whether the patient's confidentiality will be properly kept, whether the paper will be accepted by the editorial board and reviewers, or whether it will not be criticized by colleagues. When papers are to be published, there will be additional restrictions such as restriction of number of pages, so many more clinical facts have to be trimmed. Thus, the author will extract the parts that represent the patient's therapeutic process the most, like extracting cream from milk. It would be like an overall comprehensive regimen of the continuous treatment which includes the therapist's understanding and interpretations, and the patient's unconscious responses to them in the interaction of the two subjects. In that sense, clinical papers represent the refined essence of the process of the therapist-patient relationship. They brilliantly express the patient's pathological characteristics, the development of his/her unconscious world, the therapist's unconscious premises and comprehension, and other features, in much fewer pages than the numerous pages of the treatment records. Therefore, when an experienced therapist reads a clinical paper, the experience and comprehension ability of the author therapist can be grasped immediately.

The experience of publishing a clinical paper and having the author therapist's world shared and understood by other clinicians is certainly a somewhat persecutory experience where the author will be exposed to criticism. However, on the contrary, being understood and listening to sympathetic opinions will become a great force to acquire an identity as a psychoanalytic therapist.

I think that, during the period of summarizing one case for publication, something similar to dream work is occurring. As Okano states [(2)], I believe that not all expressions in the paper are distorted by neurotic censorship. There are expressions which can represent how the therapist understood the case considerably well, and there are things that can only be communicated in that way. It is considered that there also are things that can be conveyed non-verbally, but I think that they are quite limited compared to the former. There is a way to examine cases in spoken language, but the experience of expressing ourselves through publication and conveying our experiences beyond time and space is an experience regarding healthy narcissism. Publication of papers has made a great contribution to the development of psychoanalysis and will probably continue to do so. Although there may be times when therapists write and publish papers to resolve some pathological conflict, they account for only a small part, and most of the act of writing for publication is creative and developmental. It concerns a world of healthy narcissism that involves the desire of the therapist to have what they really experienced shared, understood, and respected properly by experienced seniors and colleagues, and to contribute to and make and imprint in psychoanalysis.

References

(1) Bion, Wilfred R. 1977. *Seven Servants*. New York: Jason Aronson.

(2) O'Shaughnessy, Edna. 1994. "What is a clinical fact?". *International Journal of Psychoanalysis*, Vol. 75: 939-947.

(3) Okano, Kenichiro. 1998. "The 'Rule of Abstinence' Revisited: The Clinical Significance of the 'Provision Model'". *The Japanese Journal of Psycho-analysis*, Vo.42, No. 5: 534-542. (in Japanese)

[1998. *The Japanese Journal of Psycho-analysis*, Vo.42, No. 1.]

CHAPTER 9

NEUTRALITY AND ABSTINENCE

1. Introduction

It can be said that the issue of neutrality and abstinence has historically caused great controversy. It began in old times with the dispute on "neutrality and active technique" between S. Freud and S. Ferenczi. More recently, in the United States, H. Kohut developed self-psychology, and by using the empathy theory, he shrewdly began to pursue the question of classical neutrality where the therapist with suppressed emotions is like a screen. Furthermore, recently in the United States, a situation has occurred where some clinical researchers are trying to actively utilize the therapist's self-disclosure for treatment.

On the other hand, psychoanalysts in the United Kingdom, especially the Kleinians, basically consider that Freud's neutrality and abstinence are the therapist's desirable stance, which becomes the pillar of clinical practice. They are in contrast to W. Winnicott and M. Balint and other independent school therapists who have a tendency of taking a regression-promoting therapeutic attitude that deviates slightly from the framework of neutrality.

Historically, the subtle implications in the issue of neutrality and abstinence differ in each clinical research schools, depending on treatment goals, therapeutic theories, and treatment technique theories. Some schools take a therapeutic stance that almost destroys the original neutrality.

At the end of this paper, I would like to clarify the clinical issues on neutrality of the Kleinian school, which the author was greatly influenced by. However, with regard to neutrality, various opinions have intertwined, so in order to clarify the characteristics of the Kleinian school, I feel it is necessary first to summarize the concepts and historical studies that are generally shared worldwide today.

2. Modern definition of neutrality

There are many opinions on this, but I would like to introduce those that I thinks are most generally accepted.

"*Vocabulaire de la psychanalyse*" written by J. Laplanche and J. B. Pontalis, which I will first mention, is one of the most well-compiled dictionaries that represent France. It is highly evaluated both internationally and in Japan. There, "neutrality" is described as follows:

> One of the defining characteristics of the attitude of the analyst during the treatment. The analyst must be *neutral* in respect of religious, ethical and social values—that is to say, he must not direct the treatment according to some ideal, and should abstain from counselling the patient; he must be *neutral* too as regards manifestations of transference (this rule usually being expressed by the maxim, "Do not play the patient's game"); finally, he must be *neutral* towards the discourse of the patient: in other words, he must not, *a priori*, lend a special ear to particular parts of this discourse, or read particular meanings into it, according to his theoretical preconceptions.

Secondly, R. Schafer briefly summarizes the definition of neutrality as follows:

(1) The analyst allows all conflictual material to be represented, interpreted, and worked through. He takes no sides in the consideration of these conflicts.
(2) The analyst avoids both the imposition of his own values on the patient and an unquestioning acceptance of the patient's values.
(3) The analyst is unpresumptuous as to the desirability of alternative courses of action which the patient is considering.
(4) The analyst is non-judgmental not only with respect to the patient, but also with respect to others in the patient's life.
(5) The analyst subordinates his personality to the analytic task.
(6) The analyst totally repudiates any adversarial conception of the analytic relationship.

While these definitions are the most commonly accepted, neutrality is actually being discussed in more detail by clinical researchers. This specifically stems from a critical debate on Kohut's "neutrality" in the United States. It is a criticism that the therapist's emotionless screen-like attitude at the treatment site is non-therapeutic and often anti-therapeutic as the therapist shuts his/her emotions off and disconnects the opportunities to emotionally empathize with the patient. (Kohut, etc.)

The concept of neutrality is a core concept in clinical practice; however, it seems that it has not yet reached a unified theoretical development.

Multifaceted opinions have been put forward regarding the concept of neutrality historically and in each modern school. Most of them seem to offer a unique perspective each regarding its theoretical therapeutic goals and theories of treatment techniques.

As the British Kleinians and the independent school therapists, who are strongly influenced by Klein, consider neutrality and abstinence as prerequisites for clinical activities, neutrality itself has rarely become the subject of controversy. However, the Kleinian and independent school therapists' way of involvement, their way of clinical understanding, and the actuals of their interpretations to the patients are quite specific compared to therapists of other schools. Therefore, even though it is the same neutrality, the quality of the issues of neutrality is probably subtly different depending on how the therapist is conducting actual clinical activities on the basis of its neutrality.

3. Historical transition of the concepts of neutrality and abstinence

(1) Freud's neutrality

S. Freud does not give a systematic opinion on neutrality, (Freud used the German term '*indifferenz*'. Since the English translator J. Strachey translated it as 'neutrality', 'neutrality' has become widely used.) but provides several different and important perspectives. They, in fact, imply how ambiguous the term neutrality is.

The concept of neutrality and rule of abstinence are discussed with close association. Regarding abstinence, Freud argues that the therapist must not be tempted by patients with sexual transferences and should treat them with a therapeutically appropriate distance. He also states that the therapist's basic abstinent attitude, which does not immediately try to satisfy the patient's desires, guarantees the patient's treatment motivation to continue. In this sense, Freud uses abstinence with meanings concerning the area in neutrality on the therapist's counter-transference and matters that satisfy the patient's desires.

Freud also states that, with respect to neutrality, the therapist should emotionally be in a state of coldness, or be as detached as a surgeon. Through these expressions, Freud probably wanted to emphasize the aspect of the therapist treating the patient with appropriate decisions without getting caught up in the patient's emotional vortex. Freud also wrote that the therapist should be an existence like a mirror and a screen for the patient's transferences to develop.

Seen from a somewhat different perspective, it can be said that Freud discussed the following aspects: abstinence (neutrality) as a check for the therapist's counter-transference; abstinence (neutrality) not to fulfil the patient's desire; neutrality that retains the ability to calmly judge and think about the relationship of transference and counter-transference; neutrality as the modest behaviour of the therapist who protects the patient's free associations and clearly reflects the transferences; and a neutral therapist who is not upset by the patient's transferences.

In addition, although Freud does not directly state so, things that guarantee the therapist's own "free floating attention" are also neutrality and have something in common with the stance where the therapist takes an appropriate attitude towards the patient's free association.

As mentioned above, Freud uses abstinence and neutrality in a multifaceted sense. They later developed historically, and versatile perspectives came to be advocated as in present times.

(2) Ferenczi's challenge: active technique

S. Ferenczi suggested that it may be therapeutically good for the therapist to actively satisfy a part of the desires of the patients in regression (active technique) in his theory and technique for neutrality and abstinence. He had a fierce debate with S. Freud on this, but Freud never gave way, saying that neutrality and abstinence were the therapist's core clinical attitudes for psychoanalysis.

(3) Anna Freud's concept

In regard to the concept of neutrality, among the aspects Sigmund Freud mentioned, Anna Freud especially took up the mental stance when the therapist would face the patient's mind, that is, the points regarding "free-floating attention". She considered that the therapist should be equidistant to the patient's ego, superego, and id, and that it was the most important point for the therapist's neutrality.

(4) H. Kohut's criticism on traditional neutrality techniques

Although many researchers continued to give opinions on neutrality, it was Kohut's criticism on neutrality in the United States which put forward the newest point of view. He considered that, in the United States, neutrality was distorted from its original meaning and used defensively by the therapist to prevent them from observing the patient while participating in the patient's inner world. He criticized that the therapist's emotionally-frozen neutral attitude where the therapist's feelings seemed to be coldly blocked was non-therapeutic. Kohut advocated his own unique theory of self-psychology and put forward a therapist's therapeutic attitude with an emphasis on empathy.

However, there is a problem that it is not clear whether Kohut's concept of empathy is empathy as a behaviour and action, or empathy as an intuition to understand the patient's inner world. In fact, it seems that he used the two meanings without much distinction.

4. Comprehensive theory of modern neutrality

Firstly, G. Franklin classified the above-mentioned ambiguous aspects of "neutrality" as follows. Since this is quite a comprehensive classification, it can be used as a useful basic point of view when revealing the characteristics of the British schools here.

(1) Behavioural neutrality

This is essentially a "neutrality" issue regarding Freud's rule of abstinence. In other words, it is a problem of behavioural neutrality, that is, when a patient has developed a sexual transference, the therapist must carefully check his/her counter-transference and not act to satisfy the patient's desires. In this regard, Freud refers to an objective attitude like a surgeon, a calm attitude without any therapeutic ambition, and a mirror-like attitude.

When this neutrality is used to an extreme degree, there is a risk that the therapist blocks the emotional relationship with the patient and takes a very non-therapeutic attitude. The recent critical debate on "neutrality" in the United States has to do with the problem when this behavioural neutrality is used defensively in extreme conditions.

It is said that although he advocated the above-mentioned neutral attitude, Freud himself was a very talented person who was able to interact with patients in a rich emotional manner in actual treatment.

Appropriate adherence to such behavioural neutrality and abstinence is essential in the process of encouraging patients to give free-associations and letting the patient to consciously understand their unconsciousness. Concepts such as "benevolent neutrality" (Stone, 1961) and "compassionate neutrality" (Greenson, 1958) have been proposed for this. As mentioned above, Kohut later debated an issue on neutrality which involved even the depth of the patient's personality, and stated that empathy plays a central role.

(2) Attitudinal neutrality

This is a neutrality related to the therapist's own internal attitude. Freud advocated that the therapist should have an "open mind" towards the patient, stating that analysts should not affect the patient's personality. He then argued that it was necessary for the therapist to use his/her own mind like an antenna to understand the patient's mind emotionally and intuitively. Anna Freud advocated neutrality in a sense that, since the central purpose of analytic therapy is to bring the patient's unconsciousness into consciousness, the therapist should take his/her stance "at a point equidistant from the id, the ego, and the superego". In order to do that, it is necessary to check the counter-transferences, and it is also necessary to comprehend the patient without any prejudice to understand him/her emotionally.

When the therapist misunderstands internal neutrality and goes into an extreme state where he/she freezes even his/her own emotional world, the therapist loses emotional freedom and, as a result, blocks the path to understand the patient's true emotional experiences. This is often the therapist's defensive action.

(3) Interpersonal neutrality

This is straightforwardly manifested in H. Sullivan's theory of "participant observation". In other words, he emphasized that the therapist cannot be objective with the patient, and that an interpersonal relationship always develops between them. J. Greenberg highlighted that aspect, stating that the therapist's "neutrality" is to find a subtle balance between the patient's therapist image as an old object and his/her therapist image as a new object. In this idea, it seems that there is a purpose and technique that have slightly different meanings from the original neutrality in psychoanalysis, that is, the therapist maintains "neutrality" while appropriately changing the way he/she is involved with the patient depending on the emotional state of the patient.

(4) Interactional neutrality

This is a method for the therapist to interact with the patient to fairly actively play with him/her in response to the patient's emotional state. It is related to a treatment technique where the therapist is willing to disclose him/herself. In that sense, this is a technical theory where, in a strict sense, the original neutrality has been abandoned. The pioneer of this is Ferenczi. Recently, some American analysts have advocated that true neutrality is to flexibly change the therapist's attitude according to the patient's condition. Self-disclosure is also used there as a technique.

(5) Essential neutrality

This concerns the therapist's internal attitude, especially the ability of the therapist to withstand conditions such as the agnostic of clinical materials and imperfection of interpretations since they have an aspect that they are only hypotheses. In other words, the therapist's thoughts and understandings are not always right, and he/she needs to be prepared to constantly change in response to new situations. Franklin expressly distinguishes this from attitudinal neutrality as "essential neutrality".

Next, I will show a brief summary of A. Hoffer's neutrality (1985).

(1) Neutrality is the position from which the analyst observes the world of free association.
(2) Neutrality is related to two areas. One is neutrality regarding expressions and behaviours. This is also related to abstinence, which originally encourages the patients' free associations. However, when it is overly defensively abused, it concerns issues such as feeling of indifference, unconcern, non-involvement, and detachment. The other is the issue of the therapist's power or influence on the patient. The therapist has to refrain from educational attitudes and brainwashing attitudes that instil his/her thoughts and beliefs into the patient.
(3) The influence on the patient regarding neutrality concerns the therapist's therapeutic stance. The therapist is not to take sides and be impartial and indifferent in the scientific sense of an impartial disinterest to any conflict.

Not all problems seem to be covered even with the above perspectives, but they can be a basic framework for future consideration. Both Franklin and Hoffer focus on researches in the United States. Franklin, in particular, does not discuss the Kleinian school nor the independent school of the United Kingdom, however, actually, the Kleinian school is a school that basically maintains the classical perspective on neutrality. I will discuss the details later.

5. Abstinence and ethical regulations

Abstinence is what Freud discussed as part of the issues on neutrality. It is a rule for the therapist to check his/her own counter-transference and never yield to temptation of a patient who has developed a sexual transference. This is also a warning for the possibility that the therapist may break neutrality at an important stage and disrupt the treatment itself in midway. In fact, this issue on abstinence is specifically stipulated in the ethical regulations of psychoanalytic therapy and psychoanalytic psychotherapy in terms of the therapist's social responsibilities. The ethical regulations are a text that focus on the social responsibilities of the therapist regarding abstinence. Basically, it says that the therapist must not be driven by his/her counter-transference and abuse the patient for personal desires. The ethical regulations have also become one of the most important written therapeutical structures to internally maintain the therapist's basic stance.

The therapist sometimes has difficulty maintaining the original therapist's stance because he/she is exposed to the emotional world of the patient's primitive object relations and his/her own primitive emotional world is stimulated. At that time, in addition to the spatiotemporal structure, the principle of neutrality, the principle of abstinence, and the ethical regulations play major roles in maintaining the therapeutic structure and protecting the therapist's function as a therapist. They enable the therapist to maintain a situation in which the patient understands the core of his/her true problems together with the therapist without the therapist hurting the patient who has developed an unprotected infantile primitive emotional relationship in a transference.

In fact, when abstinence and neutrality fluctuate in this way, the relationship between the therapist's counter-transference and the patient's primitive transference is often evolving the most violently, and it is often a therapeutically important turning point. At such time, the most therapeutic action the therapist can take is to maintain neutrality and strive to understand what is happening unconsciously at the treatment setting. If the therapist steps out from the neutral world and breaks the abstinence rules and ethical regulations at this most important and core timing, it means that the therapist will invade and enter into the patient's mind and re-enact the bad-parent-image which the patient projects. It will be an experience of recreating a new traumatic experience by re-enacting the relationship with the patient's traumatic parents, which will become one of the most problematic adverse reactions of treatment.

As mentioned above, abstinence has great relevance to ethical regulations. The ethical regulations are written bans for therapists at clinical settings established by the Japan Psychoanalytical Association and the Japan Psychoanalytic Society, and if they are not followed, there are penalties for certified therapists. In the case of a gross violation, the therapist may get expelled.

The basic provisions of the text include (1) obligation to keep the patient's personal information confidential, (2) prohibition of personal misuse of patient's information, (3) prohibition of sexual harassment, (4) prohibition of instilling personal beliefs and ideas such as missionary work. The therapist's external standpoint regarding social responsibility in the rules of neutrality and abstinence is clarified by them as ethical regulations, and they demonstrate one of the most fundamental clinical attitudes in psychoanalytic psychotherapy. Furthermore, the ethical regulations also play an important role as a therapeutic structure. In other words, ethical regulations, which are specified as basic principles, imply the therapeutic attitude which socially-open therapists should take, and are one of the most important guidelines that support the neutral position of the therapist at clinical settings.

Especially in psychoanalytic therapy for patients with disorders such as personality disorders, pathological object relations of such patients often occur in transferences along with strong emotions and desires. At such times, this abstinence rule and ethical regulations play important roles in protecting both the patient and the therapist from malignant acting-outs. For example, in patients who are in a state of extreme regression and exhibit strong desires and acting-outs, such abstinence rule and ethical regulations serve as a support in the background to guarantee the direction of understanding, interpreting, and resolving the dynamic meanings. If the therapist violates the abstinence rule or the ethical regulations and shows acting out in the transference of the patient's pathological object relation, driven by the patient's strong temptations and demands, it is very likely that it will be a repetition of the previous traumatic experience for the patient. By doing so, the therapist acts out as a bad object that mentally infringes on the patient, concretely reproduces the patient's traumatic object relation, and causes the patient to repeatedly experience a traumatic conflict. It is relevant to an intergenerational boundary-crossing traumatic action with the patient's parents.

6. Neutrality and abstinence in Kleinian clinical practice

Since I, the author, is deeply influenced by Klein's theory and technique, I would like to give a consideration on neutrality and discuss it in line with my experiences and the theories. The standpoint regarding neutrality of the Kleinian school and the closely-related independent school is clear. All their clinical work is carried out based on the foothold of the therapist's neutrality. In fact, since neutrality is so natural and is a major premise for their clinical activity, there are very few treatises that actively address the principles of neutrality and abstinence. Discussion is focused solely on the subject of how to understand the patient's dynamics under those conditions. For them, neutrality is the foundational position which becomes the core of their clinical activities. In fact, without this condition of neutrality, neither their clinical theories nor their therapeutic techniques can exist. However, when the meaning of neutrality is closely considered, a meaning specific to the Kleinian school is included, so I would like to describe the actual clinical activities and highlight the characteristics of Kleinian neutrality as much as possible.

Kleinian treatment goals and therapeutic techniques are related to the fact that there is a specific meaning in Kleinian neutrality. Kleinians aim to dissolve excessive pathological splitting and projective identification with interpretations to reach integration from the paranoid-schizoid position to the depressive position.

(1) Neutrality as action and behaviour

This is a matter of the therapist's attitude and behaviour. The therapist keeps on taking a passive and considerate stance of attentive listening. It is the setting and maintenance of the physical therapeutic structure such as time and space that the therapist works on actively. This is almost equivalent to classical neutrality and abstinence.

The therapist takes a neutral attitude with respect to the patient's associations and does not criticize them from his/her own point of view or try to impose or infuse his/her thoughts or ideas on the patient.

Such a neutral and abstinent therapist's attitude is considered to be the most appropriate therapist's stance to encourage free association and promote self-expression of the patient.

(2) Neutrality for the therapist him/herself

The therapist tries to adopt a specific psychic attitude when listening to the patient's associations. It is a state of mind that is expressed by words such as "free-floating attention" (S. Freud) and "no memory, no desire" (W. Bion). It is an attitude where the therapist him/herself tries to listen to the unconscious activities expressed in the patient's free associations by avoiding the bias of the mind as much as possible with respect to the patient's free association. It is also an antenna for the mind. In order to maintain such specific function of the mind, the therapist's mental neutrality is essential for the place of the mind that governs "free-floating attention" and "no memory, no desire". These are considered to be the most essential neutralities.

Next, the therapist him/herself always looks at the subtle activities of his/her own counter-transference and works to grasp the meaning of unconscious communication made by the patient's projective identification. The therapist's internal neutrality also assures the sustainability of this work. The therapist also needs a specific neutral mental attitude towards him/herself in order to understand his/her personal unresolved counter-transference activities.

The therapist selects meaningful elements and builds their unconscious meanings while he/she uses therapeutic intuition, knowledge, and experience as a whole, as he/she monitors the patient's associations and counter-transferences. Then, the therapist will internally confirm whether they are something that can be considered certain. Even in such work, there is a process where the therapist maintains a neutral viewpoint, retains a thinking space that is considered most appropriate, and understands the patient's unconsciousness.

In addition, the therapist constructs linguistic expressions which are most likely to get through to the patient and gives interpretations when the therapist considers those understandings are certain. Then, by listening to the subsequent patient's free associations, the therapist confirms the correctness of the interpretations.

As described above, the therapist takes a passive, neutral and abstinent attitude such as attentive listening in the foreground, and in the background, conducts extremely proactive and active cognitive thinking activities to understand the patient's unconscious world. What makes them work in the most appropriate state is the therapist's neutral attitude towards his/her own inner world. This therapist's neutral attitude trying to keep an appropriate distance to each of his/her mental functions is probably the most characteristic point in Kleinian neutrality. This is because Kleinian therapists probably exert their most explicit activity in regard to understanding the patient's unconscious activities and transferences, and the therapist's counter-transferences. In other words, it is because Kleinians consider that understanding the patient's here-and-now active unconscious phantasies and projective identification activities is therapeutically the most important.

7. Conclusion

I introduced the historical perspectives and the current general concepts of neutrality and abstinence. I also stated that the ethical regulations are also closely related to the issue of neutrality and play an important role in supporting the therapist's structural mental stance. Furthermore, based on a basic overview of neutrality, I explained the clinical importance of neutrality and its specific significance in the Kleinian school.

References

(1) Bion, Wilfred. 1970/1977. "Attention and Interpretation". In *Seven Servants*. New York: Jason Aronson.

(2) Britton, Ronald and Steiner, John. 1994. "Interpretation: Selected Fact or Overvalued Idea?". *International Journal of Psychoanalysis*, Vol.75: 1069-1078.
(3) Ferenczi, Sándor. 1926/1980. *Further Contributions to the Theory and Technique of Psychoanalysis*. New York: Brunner/Mazel.
(4) Franklin, Girard. 1990. "The Multiple Meaning of Neutrality". *Journal of American Psychoanalytical Association*, Vol.38: 195-220.
(5) Freud, Anna. 1936/1966. "The Ego and the Mechanisms of Defence". In *The Writings of Anna Freud,* Vol. 2. New York: International University Press.
(6) Freud, Sigmund. 1912. "Recommendations to Physicians Practicing Psychoanalysis". In *Standard Edition*, Vol. 12. London: Hogarth Press.
(7) Freud, Sigmund. 1915. "Observations on Transference Love". In *Standard Edition*, Vol. 12. London: Hogarth Press.
(8) Freud, Sigmund. 1919. "Lines of Advance in Psychoanalytic Therapy". In *Standard Edition*, Vol. 17. London: Hogarth Press.
(9) Greenberg, Jay. 1986. "Theoretical Models and the Analyst's Neutrality". *Contemporary Psychoanalysis*, Vol.22: 87-106.
(10) Hoffer, Alex. 1985. "Toward a Definition of Psychoanalytic Neutrality". *Journal of American Psychoanalytical Association*, Vol. 33: 771-795.
(11) Laplanche, Jean, and Pontalis, Jean-Bertrand. 1967. *Vocabulaire de la psychanalyse*. Paris: Presses Universitaires de France.
(12) Poland, Warren. 1984. "On the Analyst's Neutrality". *Journal of American Psychoanalytical Association*, Vol. 32: 283-299.
(13) Schachter, Joseph. 1994. "Abstinence and Neutrality: Development and Diverse Views". *International Journal of Psychoanalysis*, Vol. 75: 709-720.
(14) Segal, Hanna, and Britton, Ronald. 1981. "Interpretation and primitive psychic processes: A Kleinian View". *Psychoanalytical Inquiry*, Vol. 1: 267-277.
(15) Shapiro, Theodore. 1984. "On Neutrality". *Journal of American Psychoanalytical Association*, Vol.32: 269-282.
(16) Steiner, John. 1990. "Pathological Organizations as Obstacles to Mourning". *International Journal of Psychoanalysis*, Vol. 71: 87-94.
(17) Wolf, Ernest. 1984. "The Neutrality of the Analyst in the Analytic Situation". *Journal of American Psychoanalytical Association*, Vol. 32: 573-585.

[2002. *The Japanese Journal of Psycho-analysis*, Vol. 46, No. 2]

CHAPTER 10

UNCONSCIOUS PHANTASIES AND UNDERSTANDING OF SESSIONS

1. Development of the clinical meaning of unconscious phantasy

The complexity of the clinical meaning regarding the unconscious phantasy is one of the most intense concepts among those in psychoanalysis. It is no surprise that one of the themes chosen in the Controversies that occurred between the Kleinians and ego psychologists and a part of the analysists of the middle group in England was phantasy.

This paper will clarify the meaning of phantasy or fantasy proposed by Freud and try to elucidate the subsequent development and evolvement especially by the Kleinians. Additionally, I would like to list the characteristics of adult sessions.

Phantasy is also written as fantasy, and S. Isaacs proposed that fantasy should be used for the conscious and phantasy for the unconscious. However, it is difficult to precisely distinguish conscious from unconscious, therefore this paper standardized the term to phantasy for Isaacs and Kleinian usage here. It is common for ego psychologists and American psychoanalysts, who emphasize the viewpoint based on the formation process of phantasy due to the suppression process of Freud's daydream, to use the term fantasy.

2. Definition and development of Freud's fantasy

Descriptions on fantasy are scattered from about the Dora case [(2)], however there are no descriptions that explain it systematically. He discussed it comparatively clearly in "Formulations on the Two Principles of Mental Functioning" [(3)] and the Lecture 23 of "Introductory Lectures on Psychoanalysis" [(4)].

As seen below, Freud used one of the meanings of fantasy, which he used as a multi-faceted meaning, as his main definition. On the other hand, S. Isaacs and M. Klein paid attention to and developed the characteristics of phantasy which Freud mentioned but did not address proactively. The difference of the two is the difference of which aspect they emphasized.

Although Freud used fantasy in different places with various meanings, he defined it most clearly in "Formulations on the Two Principles of Mental Functioning" (3). He says that it is a will fulfilment that happens when a baby's instinctive wish is not fulfilled. E. Spillius (12) says that this definition is Freud's "central usage" regarding phantasy.

Freud considers about unconscious fantasy that, although there are some that are unconscious from the beginning, most of the fantasies start from conscious or preconscious daydreams and they are repressed afterwards. The fundamental motivations that create fantasies are unconscious wishes whose fulfilment is hampered. Fantasies are disguised expressions of unconscious wishes and are partial fulfilments. If such conscious or preconscious fantasies are repressed down to the unconsciousness, the patient begins to follow the primary process and they become indistinguishable from memories because they are in the unconsciousness. If daydreams are created in or repressed by the preconsciousness, they are formed following the logic of the secondary process.

In Freud's perspective, fantasies exist in the unconscious system. The basic unit that forms the unconscious system is not fantasy but an unconscious instinctual wish. According to Freud, "fantasy work" is equivalent to "dream work", and both of them transform the content of the primary unconscious wishes into a disguised form.

Freud has used fantasy containing various perspectives and in the early stage, he considered unconscious fantasy and unconscious wish as the same thing. In another place, he says that fantasy is mainly a conscious or preconscious daydream.

Furthermore, he uses fantasy with a completely different meaning in clinical practice. In the Wolfman case (5), Freud considered that the Wolfman had a fantasy of being in his mother's womb to block his father's penis when he was 1 and a half years old. Freud has not clarified whether this was a repression of what the Wolfman was originally conscious about. Also in Dora's case, many conscious fantasies are told but a part of them are unconscious fantasies (2).

Furthermore, Freud considers that some fantasies directly occur from instincts and unconsciousness, not as preconscious or conscious derivatives of unconscious wishes.

Freud mentioned about primitive fantasies in 1916. He thought they were inherited. According to Freud, concepts such as the primal scene, castration, the fantasy of being seduced correspond to this. Freud does not say that such experiences do not actually occur, but considers that such fantasies occur even if there is no external real experience that instructs such fantasies. Freud says that they "were once real occurrences in the primaeval times of the human family, and that children in their fantasies are simply filling in the gaps in individual truth with prehistoric truth". [4] This perspective is close to the thinking that when Klein's innate knowledge and Bion's "preconception" [1] coincide with experiences, concepts are formed.

As shown above, Freud used the concept of fantasy in many meanings. He was more interested in developing the meaning rather than using it as he defined it.

However, among his successors, ego psychologists and a part of the psychoanalysts of the middle group mostly inherited the "central usage", that is, the daydream theory [12]. Therefore, in the Controversies from 1943 to 1945, since a debate was held with the Kleinians based on concepts with different definitions, it just ended with both sides repeating their assertions.

3. Definitions of Klein and Isaacs, etc.

(1) Melanie Klein

Klein developed the concept of phantasy through children's play therapy from 1919. That is to say, she came to think that Freud's phantasy was the centre of psychic actions and she broadened the definition of phantasy. Klein discovered many things through children's play therapy. She stated that children were filled with conscious and unconscious phantasies and they were the centre of mental activities. According to Klein, phantasy is something endogenic, is active from birth and is a radical psychic expression of impulses and instincts. Additionally, Klein considers unconscious phantasy and unconscious thought as synonyms.

Klein mainly discovered the followings in play therapy [7]: 1) Phantasies are restrained in pathological children; 2) Phantasies about the body and the content of the mother exist universally; 3) There are various phantasies about the primal scene and the Oedipus complex; 4) Aggressive phantasy and phantasy of love are intense; 5) There is a combination of phantasies that form the depressive position (The paranoid schizoid position was added in 1946.); and 6) The development of the inner object phantasy. Klein discovered these phenomena in the rich play of children.

Later on, Klein found that the unconscious phantasy was expressed also in the behaviour and language activities of adults, and developed clinical studies on manic depressive illness (depressive position) and schizophrenia (paranoid schizoid position)[(7 (8) (9)].

(2) Susan Isaacs

In the dispute of the Controversies (a controversy that was taken place between the Kleinians vs ego psychologists and a part of the analysts of the middle group in the British Psycho-Analytical Society from 1943 to 1945), Isaacs presented an important paper "The Nature and Function of Phantasy" [(6)]. This paper is still considered as the fundamentals of the Kleinian theory of phantasy. Although short essays appear now and then, an organized theory of phantasy has not been published since her paper.

Isaacs points out the relation between Klein's theory of phantasy and Freud's concept of drive. Furthermore, she defines that the unconscious psychic process of phantasy is not secondary but primary, and is a psychic representation of the instinct. Phantasy is the same thing as what Freud gave a meaning to "representation of the instinct" and "the psychic representation of the instinctive drive".

Every individual has a continuous flow of unconscious phantasy. Whether it is normal or not is not a matter of whether the phantasy exists or not, but depends on how it is expressed and revised and how it associates with the external reality. Unconscious phantasy is the source of the unconscious mind and is an essential content that forms the original form. It is active from the earliest stage of infants and also includes the later morphology.

(1) Earliest unconscious phantasy

Klein considered that the nature of the earliest thoughts of babies was the very phantasies that are linked to physical experiences. Babies cannot visually experience phantasies so they experience them as visceral sensations and impulses, and gradually come to experience them as senses such as touch, smell, sound, taste, and sight. This is a similar idea to Freud's unconscious representation.

(2) Development theory and positions

These lead to more structured linguistic phantasies of older children and adults. Isaacs explained this from a developmental perspective. Phantasies are the basis of all experiences and they are the elements when the mind grows. Eventually, when babies show psychic development where certain states of defence such as the paranoid schizoid position and the depressive position, object relations and the group of specific anxieties are formed, unconscious phantasies exist at the basis of every element.

(3) Inner object and psychic reality

Through introjection and projection, the complex phantasy world of the inner object is created. It expands from conscious to unconscious. This, for individuals, is a certain reality and something that exerts influence for the individuals. This corresponds to what Freud called psychic reality.

(4) Words

Verbal expressions of the unconscious phantasy begin much later. Words are a means that is used unconsciously to evoke and convey the phantasies in people that exist outside.

(5) Interaction of phantasy and external reality

External reality may be understood, interpreted, and experienced by preceding phantasies. Phantasies are corrected by the experiences of external events. This interaction is the fundamentals of how the mind meets the external world and is the basis of growth and development.

(6) Phantasy and development of logical thinking

When an individual meets the external world, he/she projects the phantasy and clarifies the meaning. External reality becomes the proof or disproof of the phantasies. Logical thinking develops based on this.

(7) Relationship between defence mechanisms and phantasy

Defence mechanisms are also expressed through phantasies. Although defence is an abstract general word, in fact, it is expressed through individual phantasies. They are related to the organization of the overall personality. That is, there is a magnificent world of unconscious phantasy at the basis of all psychic activities.

(8) Development of thinking

There exist unconscious phantasies also in the back of the development of thinking. Individuals approach the reality with a foresight based on preconscious and unconscious phantasies, and constantly project phantasies into the reality. Then individuals conduct reality-testing for their phantasies and experience the reality.

(9) Psychic equilibrium and pathological organization

The composing elements of them are unconscious and conscious phantasies. The state of the psychic activities is expressed by the activities of the inner world of their phantasies. The state of fundamental anxieties and internal object relations and the state of pathological defences are based on unconscious phantasies.

(10) Contemporary Kleinians

In contemporary Kleinians, there are an emphasis on unconscious phantasies and an emphasis on the expression form of adults who actually live the infantile experiences and phantasies. In every experience, logical and non-logical phantasies are always mixed consciously and unconsciously often in unpleasant forms. It becomes therapeutically important to understand how the unconscious phantasies are expressed in symbolic contents, and interpret them focusing on how the patient manages to live in the psychoanalytic sessions.

4. Sessions and unconscious phantasies

As shown above, individual's psychic inner structure and activities are premised on unconscious phantasies and preconscious phantasies. As the individuals grow from early infancy to childhood, puberty, adolescence and adulthood, the experience world becomes structured to a more grown state from a primitive state. However, in the back, there is a world of unconscious phantasy that supports a psychic world further differentiated from the phantasies in a more primitive state.

It is viewed that even the lowermost layer of the unconscious phantasy is linked to symbols and linguistic functions in the upper layers, and there are times when they are expressed extremely complicatedly even in the conscious expressions. In the level of individuals who have a background of moderate personality disorder like Ms. C, who will be introduced in this paper, unconscious phantasies presumably act as a meaningful connection of the inner object relation. This means that unconscious phantasies are in a state where the meanings are linked as anxieties, defences and object relations in the paranoid-schizoid position and the depressive position. Primitive phantasies that become the basis of them exist as a foundation in the lower layers further under those unconscious inner worlds. They may be the most primitive unconscious phantasies in the world which corresponds to the foundation of the mind, which Bion expressed as the alpha function's formation process; from sense impressions to alpha elements [(1)].

Adult patients with disorders such as psychosis and neurosis, or borderline cases are patients with active unconscious phantasies of a level formed in a kind of ramified state basically because of objects whose inner object relations are interrelated. It is considered that a mental function that links to the symbolic world and links from the unconscious thoughts to the conscious thoughts, or from the unconscious verbal world to the conscious verbal world is in action. This may be why we therapists can trace back to the active state of the unconscious phantasies from the conscious verbal associations of adult patients and verbally grasp and deliver them to the patients themselves.

In the connection from this primitive level of unconscious phantasy to the level of abstract thoughts of adults, it is considered that there lies a level of primitive unconscious phantasy in the basic part of the innermost of the mind. On top of that, there evolves an organized world of inner object relations such as the paranoid-schizoid position and the depression position, an active layer that expresses them with means such as dreams, and furthermore, a world of advanced psychic functions including abstract thoughts, symbols, and verbal expressions. It is not an easy work to understand the developmental involvement of the unconscious phantasy regarding the continuity. It can be said that Bion tried to express the formal state of unconscious phantasies from a primitive level to a level of abstract thoughts by Grid (1).

Although therapy sessions are based on verbal expression with free association in a certain therapeutic structure, non-verbal expressions such as behaviour, voice inflection, acting-in and acting-out exist simultaneously. It is considered that unconscious phantasies are active in all the above stated stages. It may be that unconscious phantasies of the various stages are present there as respective fundamental existences in the unconsciousness to the preconsciousness. They include the early phantasies that represent the extremely primitive instinct initiative, the world of object relations that is developmentally growing from the paranoid-schizoid position to the depressive position, and unconscious phantasies underlying in the relatively later psychic function ranging from phantasies to verbal expressions, abstraction, symbols, and defence mechanisms. A world of the session's conscious phantasies including conscious verbal expressions, dreams and fantasies is established on the foundation of those unconscious phantasies.

In adult therapy, a story world of a certain image is developed by expressions in sessions conducted with free associations. It is considered to be basically the same as the description of the story developed in children's play. However, in the case of adults, it is not easy to understand the movement of the unconscious phantasies because various elements, such as the state of anxiety, the position of development, complex defence mechanisms, abstract function and thinking function, intertwine. On the other hand, in the case of children's play, the world of the children's unconscious phantasies is in action right near conscious play like opencast mining, while the rich world of phantasies and the almost primitive defences are active unsystematically (7).

The therapist attentively listening to the adult sessions make certain considerations: Which part of the unconscious mind is expressed? Which position? What are the characteristics of the anxiety? What are the expressions of the symbolic function and defence mechanisms? What kind of materials were used to express them? In what form, that is, verbal expressions, acting-out, dreams or acting-in, are they expressed? Compared to the direct rich expressions of children' play, the characteristics of adult sessions are that their conscious expressions are distorted, split-off, indirect, and fragmented. Psychic functions and actions of all the developmental stages are chaotically mixed there and unconscious phantasies are not often directly expressed.

The fundamentals of treatment for the therapist are to clarify the unconscious and preconscious themes of such adult sessions and to reveal and interpret the fundamental anxieties, defence mechanisms and transferences lurking in the themes.

Dreams are a part of the unconscious phantasies expressed by imagination during sleep, and are representatives of something that vividly expresses the theme of that point [(11)]. Complex processes such as defensive thinking and abstraction intervene also in the reporting of daily events and experiences in sessions, and it is often the case that anxiety and infantile themes are covered with many layers. Frequently, important themes are expressed in the selection of the subject and the development of the story, in the same manner as dreams.

5. Case presentation

Case Patient

The patient was Ms. C, a woman in her 30s.

Main complaints

Depersonalization, repetition of depressive attacks, checking compulsion (gas cocks, keys), intense feeling of self-insufficiency

Her brother has an impulsive emotionally unstable personality.

Psychoanalysis was conducted 3 times a week using the couch.

Ms. C reported a dream in the first session that "she had a deformity in her neck but her mother says there was no need to worry" and an additional dream that "a burglar was peeping into her room a few times". As Freud clarified, dreams are expressions of dream thoughts associating distortion of expressions such as symbols, displacement and condensation of the unconscious motivations and anxieties. From a perspective of the phantasy theory, dreams indirectly express a part of the unconscious phantasy which is currently in action.

The first dream represents the patient's worries and anxieties regarding the significance of her own disease and expresses a persecutory experience which is an invasion into her own body. It should be her mother who discovers her disease and takes care of her and leads her to cure. However, her mother cannot help the patient because she does not realize the deformity. The dream expressed not only a maternal aspect of the therapist (displacement and symbols), but also the patient's anxiety and doubt against the unknown therapist upon starting therapy, and the early transference to the therapist as an object that has a possibility of rescuing her.

Additionally, as for the dream where the burglar peeped into the patient's room, the patient's anxiety is a persecutory anxiety that she would be peeped into her mind. The dream expresses her fear that the content of her mind and body would be stolen by the burglar. These are also expressions of an unconscious phantasy, and the persecutory invasive aspect of the therapist is expressed by displacement and symbols. Dreams can brilliantly express this unconscious situation.

When unconscious phantasies are expressed as dreams, phenomena such as symbols, displacement, and condensation come into operation and various people and matters appear in the iconic expressions. This is one of the manifestations of defence. The therapist tries to read the indirect expressions and grasp a small part of the patient's unconscious phantasy. It is also an expression of the transference and an expression of the patient's fundamental anxiety, too. Furthermore, when a story is composed, thoughts are in action and verbal expressions are involved too.

As stated above, every psychic function, such as individual unconscious phantasies, the state of anxiety and positions, state of defence, thoughts, verbal expressions, and symbolic function, are simultaneously in action in the patient's reporting of dream.

What the therapist aims there is to focus on and understand matters including the fundamental anxieties, the characteristics of the developmental stage (position), the therapist image and the transference relation expressed with symbols and displacement, and the association between the countertransference and the content of the dreams. Then the therapist verbalizes mainly the state of the anxiety and the transference to the therapist and conveys them to the patient as interpretations.

In such a process, the therapist makes full use of his/her knowledge and ability to understand, which he/she acquired with his/her specific intuitive ability, and through experience, and conveys the content of the understandings he/she obtained to the patient. Language is used at that time. The role of language is to convey the phantasies and thoughts of the individuals to others. It is expected that the listener will picture almost similar phantasies and thoughts in his/her mind with the common language.

In actual sessions, I, the therapist, gave the following interpretation: "Upon starting therapy, the problems the patient has are serious and severe but your mother in your dream is too insensitive to notice them. Similarly,

I guess you are worried that I, the therapist, also will not realize them and will not pay any serious attention to them. You are also worried that I will peep into your mind and just steal your precious things and will not help you."

Ms. C replied to this, "I always complain to my mother about how she treats my brother." Even in such associations, the patient has thoughts of unconscious phantasies and tells conscious matters related to them. What she reports as daily matters also have unconscious motivations for adopting the expression and are related to the unconscious phantasies. The therapist told her, "By saying so, you are also complaining about how your mother treats you." The therapist continued, "I think you are worried whether I, the therapist, will treat you properly and provide treatment for you." A partial replacement can be seen here where the mother is the therapist and the younger brother is the patient. The patient manifests her anxieties towards treatment and associations regarding the therapist with expressions like some types of metaphors or hidden messages, that is, with an intervention of subtle defence mechanisms, to express the theme.

Here, the experience world of the patient's earliest primitive unconscious phantasy reacted to the reality experience that we would start therapy, which is expressed as dreams and conscious fantasies. The therapist retrospectively traces back the patient's conscious verbal expressions and reaches to a part of the unconscious phantasy which is the infantile primitive object relation at the bottom of the them. Then, the therapist seeks what kind of experiences the patient is having in that world about the therapy and about the therapist, and conveys them as interpretations to the patient who is having the associations.

Returning to the clinical case, Ms. C additionally told me, "I sometimes had a fantasy that a witch would come out from the cupboard." This association too is one of the tangled expressions of the unconscious phantasy that chose the theme. Although this is a day dream, it is a tangled expression of the unconscious phantasy just like dreams. In this manner, patients who can verbally express their fantasies and thoughts with free association are conducting multiple mental activities simultaneously, and can express their fantasies and stories related to unconscious phantasies with language by interplaying versatile defence mechanisms and anxieties and can convey them to the therapist.

Klein discovered that the method of dream interpretation developed by Freud could also be applied to the understanding of the reports of patients' *waking conscious* associations and fantasies. This is an application of the children's play therapy to the understanding of the free-association sessions of adult patients. This is one of the most important discoveries among the many discoveries made by Klein, which brought about an innovative revolution to contemporary psychoanalysis.

The therapist gave an interpretation, "The cupboard is the world of your mother and expresses the fearsome world which your witch-like mother appears from. It also represents the just-begun therapeutic site. It is related to your fear that the existence of me the therapist might actually have a fearsome, weird aspect that threatens you." In this way, Ms. C often expressed her fear and anxieties regarding the start of treatment with dreams and associations.

In the following session, Ms. C said, "Something is wrong. I spill coffee and miss my step on the stairs." The therapist asked her, "Do you have a load on your mind?", and she replied, "My father is a really fearsome person and I get violently scorched if I make a blunder in even the slightest terms." She added, "My father is a scary person. He would sudden become angry and use violence against me, and when he has small troubles while driving, he would kick the other person's car or yell at him/her. He also seems to have charisma and deflates others with odd logics." By saying so, Ms. C conveyed to me that it was one of her biggest problems to have been hurt in the many experiences with such a father, and it was a task she would have to face in the upcoming treatment. She also implied the transference relationship with the therapist. The therapist gave an interpretation, "I guess you are being timid wondering what to do if I, the therapist, was such a persecutory scary existence like your father. And, I think you are worried upon starting treatment that I may become mad if you cannot give good associations and make a mess even in the slightest terms."

In the following session, Ms. C said very worriedly, "I do not want to think about my sick relatives. I don't want to expose my point of weakness. I want to sort out my feelings," and "My father is the real problem and my brother is a problem, it is not my problem." The therapist told her, "I guess that you are getting concerned that if you talk about yourself freely, it may turn out that you have to responsibly solve the serious problems of all the members of your family, and have a feeling that you will encounter difficulty."

In addition, Ms. C said, "My aunt is trying to switch blames on our family about the problem of my elder male psychotic cousin. Although the aunt is one of the decent people among my relatives, when I went to stay at her house the other day, she charged me a bath fee so she is not decent." The therapist mentioned about the matter of the treatment fee and interpreted, "I think you are suspicious that I am actually just after money and cannot understand you properly and helping you is secondary."

In the following session, Ms. C said that in here dream, "A man came into my room and replaced the refrigerator and the washing machine. There is no drain so the washing machine was flooded." Ms. C had associations about men including a cold man who she had slept with but that was all to it, and a man who would make prank calls.

The therapist considered that this dream represented the transference to the therapist and gave an interpretation, "The man represents the therapist's untrustworthy aspect that makes bad use of Ms. C and also expresses the therapist who enjoys using, pranking and hurting Ms. C." Furthermore, this dream expressed that the patient could not remove her distrust, fear, and cautiousness against the therapist at this early period of treatment. In addition, the therapist interpreted, "The refrigerator is something that stores the patient's unsettled mind, and the washing machine contains a meaning of the treatment that washes your mind. I guess you are worried whether I am a terrible therapist who makes a blunder like changing just the places of those machines and ruins your heart." Ms. C said anxiously, "I wonder if you see through everything like that and if you are a scary person. I want to know what kind of person you are and where you come from."

In such actual sessions, there is a process of understanding the activities of the unconscious phantasies and grasping the states of transference and defence. Collectively, it can be said that there are the following perspectives in the background.

(1) Adults' free association

Free association of adults is equal to children's play and expresses the unconscious phantasy. Compared to children's play, the content of adults' free association is extremely complex because of aspects such as abstract expressions, guise of rational thinking and activity of the sophisticated defence mechanisms. However, what is important is that the expression of unconscious phantasies is conducted in twists and turns.

(2) The subject and theme of the topic the patient chose

The therapist will understand the unconscious motivation why the patient chose the material. Which material the therapist chooses to understand the dynamics at that point is based on training and experience, and his/her comprehensive ability including his/her thinking ability and his/her therapeutic intuitive ability. The correctness and the fallacy can be judged by the development of associations and the progress of the patients' self-understanding in the therapeutic course. Additionally, the intuitive judgment of a third party's perspective such as supervision and study meetings are useful. At any rate, it is something with a relative characteristic of mutual cognition in human communication. At all times, only the relative correctness can be assumed. The difficulty of psychoanalytic clinical practice lies here.

(3) Main clinical viewpoints of the therapist

As for main clinical viewpoints, the therapist interpreted matters such as anxiety, defence, and characteristics of the inner object relation by paying attention to the followings: 1) what the associations that implied Ms. C's true anxiety and fear were like, 2) how the defences such as introjection and projective identification are functioning, 3) how the symbolic function is acting, 4) what the unconscious transference to the therapist is like, and 5) what the countertransference is like.

6. Conclusion

This paper discussed the complexity and universality of unconscious phantasy. In addition, it explained how unconscious phantasies are expressed in adult case sessions. They are covered with complex adult defence mechanisms, abstraction and ambiguity of language and become distorted and vague. The therapist distinguishes various phenomena such as conflict, defence, and abstraction among the associations in the sessions and tries to approach the action of the phantasies related to the core anxiety and pain.

References

(1) Bion, Wilfred Ruprecht. 1963. *Elements of Psychoanalysis*. London: Heinemann.

(2) Freud, Sigmund. 1905. "Fragment of Analysis of a Case of Hysteria". In *Standard Edition*, Vol. 7. London: Hogarth Press.

(3) Freud, Sigmund. 1911. "Formulations on the Two Principles of Mental Functioning". In *Standard Edition*, Vol. 12. London: Hogarth Press.

(4) Freud, Sigmund. 1916-1917. "Introductory Lectures on Psychoanalysis". In *Standard Edition*, Vol. 15-16. London: Hogarth Press.

(5) Freud, Sigmund. 1918. "From the History of an Infantile Neurosis". In *Standard Edition*, Vol. 17. London: Hogarth Press.

(6) Isaacs, Susan. 1948. "The Nature and Function of Phantasy". *International Journal of Psychoanalysis*, Vol. 29: 73-97.

(7) Klein, Melanie. 1932/1975: "Psychoanalysis of Children". In *The Writings of Melanie Klein*, Vol. 1. London: Hogarth.

(8) Klein, Melanie. 1935/1975. "A Contribution to the Psychogenesis of Manic-Depressive States". In *The Writings of Melanie Klein*, Vol. 1. London: Hogarth.
(9) Klein, Melanie. 1940/1975. "Mourning and its Relation to Manic-Depressive States". In *The Writings of Melanie Klein*, Vol, 1. London: Hogarth Press.
(10) Klein, Melanie.1946/1975. "Notes on Some Schizoid Mechanisms". In *The Writings of Melanie Klein*, Vol. 3. London: Hogarth Press.
(11) Segal, Hanna. 1991. *Dream, Phantasy and Art*. London: Routledge.
(12) Spillius, Elizabeth. 2001. "Freud and Klein on the Concept of Phantasy". *International Journal of Psychoanalysis*, Vol. 82: 361-373.
(13) Steiner, Riccardo. 2003. "Introduction". In *Unconscious Phantasy*, edited by Riccardo Steiner, 1-66. London: Routledge.

[2012. *The Japanese Journal of Psycho-analysis*, Vol. 53, No. 4]

CHAPTER 11

THE MECHANISM AND GOAL OF TREATMENT: FROM A KLEINIAN PERSPECTIVE

1. Introduction

The subject of this paper "The Mechanism and Goal of Treatment" includes extremely wide-ranging problems. In the background, there lies issues regarding the therapeutic goal, the understanding of the therapeutic process and the termination of treatment. Simply put, the purpose of treatment is not only the general health recovery but also achievement of therapeutic goals such as solving the patient's inner conflict or promoting development of the patient's mentality based on the therapeutic mechanism the therapist stands on. As for the former, the barometers are generally improvement of symptoms, improvement of work or social function or the possibility of getting a job or entering a school.

However, from the perspective of psychoanalytical therapists, it is generally considered that even though the symptoms show general improvement, if the patient's inner mental problems are not solved, the patient has not improved in the true sense. This is also related to the issue of transference cure or the situation called escape towards health. In such a situation, it is often the case that most of the symptoms disappear, however, when treatment is terminated because both the patient and the therapist mistake that the patient is cured, most of the patients suffer a relapse.

The therapeutic mechanism and the therapeutic goal are largely dependent on the psychoanalyst's theoretical perspective. There is an aspect where the therapist defines the therapeutic approach and technique, the method to understand the therapeutic process, and the therapeutic goal according to how he/she understands the inner mental pathology of the patient.

In this paper I would like to first refer to Freud's fundamental theoretical perspective and therapeutic mechanism and introduce the Kleinian theoretical development up to today and then its therapeutic mechanism and goal. Thereafter, I would like to present a case and add considerations about the therapeutic mechanism and the therapeutic goal.

2. Sigmund Freud's Theory of Neurosis and the Therapeutic Mechanism and Therapeutic Goal

a The Damming Up of Libido Theory and the Therapeutic Mechanism

Freud's early theory of neurosis stated that "Mental illness results from sexual suppression." Therefore, the mechanism and goal of treatment was to support the patients to discharge sexual love from such suppression in a satisfying way.

b The Topographical Theory and the Therapeutic Mechanism

Next, Freud divided human mentality into consciousness, preconsciousness and unconsciousness and regarded that the conflict in-between the impulse and drive in the unconsciousness and the requirements of reality were the core of neurosis. Therefore, Freud set "making the unconsciousness conscious" as the centre of the therapeutic mechanism and goal. To accomplish this, he regarded that handling resistance adequately in treatment was an important therapeutic technique.

c The Structural Theory and the Therapeutic Mechanism

Furthermore, after Freud introduced the theory of structure of ego, super-ego and id in 1923, he began to consider that the core of neurosis was a result where the ego could not adequately adjust the desire of super-ego and id and the requirements from the outer world. Therefore, it became important as a therapeutic mechanism and became the therapeutic goal to adequately alleviate the relationship of ego and super-ego and the relation of ego and id. Freud especially focused on the importance of the relationship of id and ego and has left a famous phase "Where id is, let ego be."

To realize these in actual treatment, Freud thought that not only the handling of resistance but also interpretation of the transference and the patients' understanding of them through their "insight" were important in transference neurosis. In other words, from the therapists' standpoint, the primary therapeutic goal is that the therapist can provide therapeutic intervention so that such therapeutic mechanism would fundamentally operate and that the patients can subsequently achieve self-understanding of them through "insight".

Subsequently to Freud, many analysts have stated about the mechanism and goal of treatment, however basically they are considerations from Freud's structure theory standpoint.

3. The Kleinian Therapeutic Mechanism and Goal

Since I have strongly been influenced by the Kleinian school, I would like to give a consideration on the therapeutic mechanism and goal from a Kleinian perspective. The Kleinian therapeutic mechanism, therapeutic goal and barometer of therapeutic efficacy are naturally based on the theory and pathology of the mind. From the therapist's perspective, the biggest goal of treatment is an integrated transition from the paranoid-schizoid position towards the depressive position. Therefore, it is most important for the therapeutic mechanism to restore into the self the world of the inner object imago and self imago which have been split off by primitive defence mechanisms such as splitting, projective identification and denial. It is considered that the work where the therapist understands the world which is split off into the patient's unconsciousness or outer others due to such defence mechanisms, through the content of free-associations or acting-outs, or the relationship of transference/countertransference, and interprets those understandings to the patients will bring about a therapeutically important inner integration.

Wilfred Bion explained this process with the model of container/contained. When a transference situation occurs where the patient (baby) splits off the part of self and the inner object which cannot be integrated and projectively identifies with the outer world, the therapist (the mother), the therapist (mother) who was introjected the split-off part (transference) experiences normal counter-transference emotions or ideas conveyed by a verbally-told inner imaginary world or nonverbal communication. By synthesizing and integrating them, the therapist (mother) understands the meaning of the activity of the patient's (baby's) split-off unconscious inner world and conveys the interpretations back to the patient. In this way, the therapist (mother) plays an important role as the function of a container. This means that the function of the container includes not only maintenance of the therapeutic structure or supportive care for the patients but also the proactive attitude and directivity of the therapist who understands and interprets the patient's primitive communication. At actual therapeutic sites, the therapist concentrates on understanding a part of the unconscious world which the patient conveys through free association, his/her attitude or atmosphere or acting out, and integrating them to discover the world of the meaning. In daily sessions, the therapist repeats therapeutic work where he/she interprets these unconscious meanings with words which the patient can understand. This work itself is related to the important function of the container.

The patients themselves have felt from their childhood that they could not handle these painful experiences. Therefore, they often have formed an organized defence organization against the fact that they will become aware of those object relations and that they will return to them. This is mostly seen in patients with severe pathological personality problems. The representative theories are personality theories such as H. Rosenfeld's "narcissistic organization" and J. Steiner's "pathological organization".

The latter "pathological organization" is a typical modern Kleinian theory of pathological personality. According to Steiner, it is a pathological third position: while the healthy part of self has a tendency to trust and be dependent on the therapist and tries to develop, this pathological third position has a tendency to give a pathological warning, strongly attack such healthy part of self and stubbornly resist change. Furthermore, the inner world of the pathological organization is founded on fragmentary introjection and amalgamation of the bad objects and self that plunged the self into frustration. It is filled with persecutory anxiety and depressive anxiety which is composed of a world of pathological part object relations. A sado-masochistic object relation is active there and a pervasive object relation and an addictive object relation with destructivity are prominent. If they are strong, they play a big role in forming a severe pathological personality.

The therapist finds out and interprets the indications of the patient's split-off world while understanding such mechanism. The therapist heads towards the therapeutic goal where the patient becomes aware of them and integrates the depressive position.

In this process, the patient becomes aware that he/she had denied he/she had suffered from an ambivalent relation with the object, that while he/she had directed his/her hate, anger or aggression at such object on the other hand he/she was dependent on it, and that he/she would have a painful experience or a pathological feeling of guilt when he/she loses it. In this process, the patient gradually comes to be able to develop his/her thought and symbolic function.

In this process, the conflicting aspect of the split-off object becomes clear so the patient has no other choice but to become aware of his/her various complaints, painful experiences or aggression and excessive guilt against the object. This is extremely painful for the patient him/herself and brings about hurt and anxiety, which become a strong force to prevent the treatment to develop. They also often function as intense pathological organizations and the patient tries to get his/her revenge on the fact that he/she was treated unjustly and tends to identify with the attacker or show self-destructive actions. It is often the case that the therapist is involved in the world of the pathological object relation and is made to play a role to strengthen it.

These are therapeutic theories as well as therapeutic mechanisms and therapeutic goals based on the Kleinian pathological personality theory. In parallel with the general therapeutic goal where the patient's symptoms improve and the social function improves, the therapist evaluates to what degree the patient was able to achieved the above-mentioned inner changes and uses it as criteria to judge whether the therapeutic goal has been achieved and when to terminate therapy.

4. Case

I would like to present a case where the patient improved due to the therapist's understanding and interpretation of her split-off world which she expressed through free-association, acting-out, projective identification and many dreams.

Case

The case patient M was a housewife in her 40s. The diagnosis was chronic depression. In the background, there was a tendency of a dependent narcissistic personality. She had a salaried-worker husband, an elementary school daughter and son. Four years before the year she came for consultation, a female friend of M, whom she had a dependent relationship with, died because of cerebral tumour. This triggered M to become depressive and since then she has received various treatments for depression such as anti-depressants dosing and electroshock, however she had not improved. Her regular physician recommended her to get pregnant as she might get better, however she had a miscarriage and the depression became worse. M could hardly do the household chores and mostly stayed lied down for several years and her depressive state still continued. M's regular physician recommended her to receive psychoanalytical psychotherapy.

M lived apart from her parents for the first time when she entered university (at the age of 18). However, she suffered from the fear of loneliness and had extreme anxiety attacks and fell into depression. At that time, she consulted a religious worker and somehow got back on her feet and returned to university in a few months.

M's mother lost her parents when she was a child. She received higher education with a strong will and brought M up with strict discipline. When M was very young child, her mother was hospitalized for 6 months due to cancer and underwent a surgical procedure. M was left at her aunt's house.

During the 6 months, M did not gain any weight and when her mother came to get her after she was discharged from hospital, M said she did not recognize her mother.

M's father was also a person who lost his parents when he was a child and was brought up by his relatives. He could not have affectionate interactions and was engaged in work. He did not try to interact with his family, therefore his relationship with M was tenuous.

Her older sister rebelled against her mother's dominant strict discipline from about adolescence so she was always fighting with her mother. M was afraid of her mother so she behaved herself and spent her childhood being obedient to her mother's strict requirements.

Therapeutic Process

Treatment was conducted 3 times a week on the couch.

(1) The 1st period (The first 6 months)

In the early stage of treatment, M had an intense suspicion against the therapist and showed a strong anxiety to be near to the therapist. However, she gradually reacted to the therapist's interpretations on her anxiety and began to show an attitude to approach the therapist after she talked about "a news on television where a person very alike the therapist saved the victims". In free association, although it was indirect, M expressed the world related to her unconscious phantasy well through displacement and the symbolic function. Therefore, in regard to understanding much of the unconscious split-off world, the therapist was able to understand the abundant activities of the patient's split-off inner world through the symbolized expressions based on her verbal expressions. For example, M told the therapist stories that her choice of her husband might have been wrong, that her husband did not accompany M to a funeral and she was the only one without a partner. Furthermore, she said that a doctor she knew said she would give ballet shoes to M's daughter but the doctor forgot and did not keep her promise. These include symbolic expressions which express a sense of distrust and anxiety about the choice of the therapist, that her true conflictive problem was object loss. They further expressed her distrust and anxiety that the therapist might not support her mourning work nor give her what she needed or something to let her stand on her feet and take on a life of her own, as the therapist promised.

While we were talking about the anxieties of the introduction period, M told the therapist that she took the plunge and bought a new plant saying, "I don't know how to take care of it and feel like I am having an adventure." This was an manifestation of her mind that she would like to accept the therapeutic experiences she had in the relationship with the therapist and do something but did not know what to do. When the therapist interpreted this, M said "I have begun to think that you might understand and help me." As seen from above, M was good at verbal expressions and was a person who could express the world of her preconscious split-off inner object relation with symbolic expressions and acting-outs.

Thereafter, M said "My daughter has suddenly gone nuts. She kept on crying and crawled saying she was born today. What's the matter with her? I should have treated her with more affection, it's too late." The therapist interpreted that "M was projecting her own baby part into her daughter and her daughter was expressing that emotion by acting-out so M was able to see herself through that." Furthermore, M said "These days, my hands move automatically so I am writing a lot in my own room. When I read it, I became so frightened that I sealed and locked it, so it is all right now." She then said something nonsensical, "But I think you can read it," and fell into a confused state. The therapist had a strong anxiety that M might have fell into a psychotic state. However, M came to the next session on time and said "I had a talk with my husband and was thinking about my future self." and showed her strength of self that she could somehow overcome the confused state she was in in the last session. The therapist was anxious that she might psychotically fall apart, therefore he was relieved.

When the therapist told M about his vacation later, she suddenly got in a bad mood and recalled that when she was 2 years old her mother left her behind. Then M began to say "I am 2 years old now. My body has become small and my breathing and also my hands are those of the 2-year-old me." When the end of the session came, M stretched her hand out and asked the therapist to help her up. M was extremely angry against the therapist because he did not try to help her up and she blew her top at her family after she went home. Furthermore, just before the therapist's vacation, M said "Since a symbol of God appeared at my bedside, I have been saved so I am all right even if I don't come to therapy." On the other hand, she told stories about her cousin who made a suicide attempt, about a woman who committed suicide after killing her parents and that she had her cat killed at a public health centre. Through these stories, she expressed that she had a murderous anger and a strong abandonment fear related to death against the brief separation with the therapist.

The characteristics of such M's object relation in the transference relationship was that it was composed of ambivalence between a pathological, unsolved abandonment fear and an intense dependence in the depressive position, and ambivalence between intense anger, depression, persecutory sense of guilt and impulse of self-punishment against the object loss. This is what Klein clearly described as the pathological state of the depressive position which expresses that the pathological core of psychogenic depression is in the patient's split-off pathological depressive position.

The role of the therapist was to interpret what the therapist understood about the split-off unconscious world which M indirectly symbolically expressed mainly through such daily topics and acting-outs. Through the therapist's interpretations, M became aware of and integrated what she had split off until then. This work is an important therapeutic mechanism and the core of the therapeutic process.

(2) The 2nd Period (6 to 12 months)

From this period, M began to colourfully and abundantly report symbolic associations and dreams. For example, in the session after the holiday, M talked about the winter jacket which her mother gave her. M was given the jacket about when her mother died 10 years ago. Her mother had not washed it so it was not clean. M said, "I washed the jacket during the holidays but the waterproofing had worn off so I think I can't wear it anymore." This symbolically indicated that during the holidays M tried to get back under the aegis of her inner mother, however, on the other hand she also thought she wanted to cleanly dispose of and sort out her mother's legacy. M did so symbolically by washing it, however in return, it meant that she could not receive the stained aegis of her mother anymore. This washing means treatment and expresses that if M received treatment she felt that she would lose her mother's protection. Furthermore, her mother's aegis was dirty and it was an unpleasant thing for M. As seen above, M began to be able to richly express the ambivalent relationship with her mother in the transference relation with the therapist.

By that time, M told critical remarks and was rebellious against her mother. Associations where M enjoyed the free liberated world with the therapist and the world of intense abandonment fear and the fear of death when M tried to separate from and become independent of the persecutory mother could be seen in turns. M then reported the following dream. "I was working at my working place and the timetable was not in order so I did not know which classroom I had to go. Another female staff came and said such a timetable is unnecessary and enjoyed ripping and scattering it." M said that the female staff was a free, independent senior associate who lived on her own will whom M respected a lot. This expressed that M herself was rebellious against her mother's world where her mother required strict punctuality from M and that M had a desire to be freed. It also expressed her rebellion against the therapist's strictness that he only met her at the scheduled time. Additionally, M was expressing that she wanted to live her life freely like her senior associate. When the therapist interpreted this to M she nodded as she accepted the interpretation.

From this period, M's depressive state rapidly improved and she began to go out with her daughter and play with her in the park.

However, on the other hand, M reported that her daughter had a dream. "When I (M's daughter) was at home, a monster appeared so I ran away. I forgot to put my shoes on so I went back. I was caught and eaten up and was buried in a grave." M reported that this dream was reported by her daughter, however projective identification was actively performed between M and her daughter and M's part of dream activity was projectively identified into her daughter. Therefore, it could be considered that the dream M's daughter had was equal to the dream M had and it meant that the boundary between them was in an ambiguous state. The therapist interpreted, "This dream was a dream which M's alter ego, her daughter, had for M because M had projectively identified a part of her self into her daughter." Thus, the therapist decided to handle this dream equally to a dream which M had. It can be considered that this dream expressed that M criticized and rebelled against her mother's world and was trying to freely enjoy herself in the world with the therapist, however at the same time, she was having an inner experience where she was attacked by her monstrous persecutory mother who did not allow her to. M tried to escape; however, she was not ready enough to be independent so she went back to her house which is her very mother. Then she is eaten and introjected by the monster (her mother) and is buried in the world of the graveyard where her mother is dead. This dream expresses M's intense fear of object loss, her persecutory anxiety and persecutory feeling of guilt. This was actually an object relation which was routinely enacted in reality between M and her daughter.

In the next session, M told the following dream of her own. "When I was enjoying my bicycle ride in town, there was a wall. Two men lifted me and my bicycle up and put me down on the other side. However, there was another high wall so, out of necessity, I had them help me back to the original place." It seems that this dream expresses that M tried to escape from her mother's world with the help of two men, the therapist and her administrative doctor, however she returned to it as she found that it was impossible. Again, M accepted this interpretation with understanding.

By this period, clinically, M's depressive state had improved and she had come to be able to live her daily life normally. However, the therapist considered that this had an aspect of the so-called transference cure and that M was in the stage where she was just beginning to see the world of a conflictive relationship with the object. M sometimes said, "I have become quite well so I think treatment is not necessary anymore. My family also says that I don't have to come anymore." However, from the perspective of the therapeutic treatment, the therapist considered this as a sign that M was trying to avoid touching the world of the true conflictive inner object relation. Actually, in the therapeutic process of psychoanalytical psychotherapy, this kind of improvement of clinical symptoms are often seen, however, it is a transference cure or avoidance towards health. In fact, it is often the case that the patient's most painful and difficult-to-touch inner world is approaching.

(3) The 3rd Period (1 year to 2 and a half years (termination))

Thereafter, M's symptom did not aggravate and she began to work part-time after a year from the start of treatment. The therapist consistently focused on how M could become aware of the painful world of object relation with the inner object and how she could integrate it. Therefore, the therapist did not consider that the therapeutic process had substantially proceeded just by M's symptomatic and overall improvement. There was a long period where M expressed herself through many dreams, symbolic expressions and acting-outs and the therapist interpreted the unconscious meanings of them. Practicing this working-through is important for treatment. The true termination of treatment will arrive when not only the patient's clinical symptoms have improved but also the patient's conflictive split-off world is made aware of and integrated through the understanding of the transference relation to the therapist brought about by this working-through.

After a year from the start of treatment, M gave abundant associations and reported many dreams. M took good care of the plant in the treatment room and associated sadly that she never even had as much freedom as the plant. She then said, "My mother strictly regulated me so my true desires have never been satisfied nor have I been dependent on someone at ease." She continued that the regulation was gradually coming off because of treatment.

Around that time, M had the following dream: "I was taking an examination. I prepared for only 2 subjects but the teacher told me to take 3 subjects. It was too late." In regard to this, the therapist interpreted that what M had not prepared for was the termination of treatment. Then M reported the following dream: "You were in the bed room of my house. I was in the toilet listening to your conversation. Then you began to play the piano. I thought you were good but I felt that I shouldn't listen. A family whose daughter died because she was using narcotic drugs was having a farewell party downstairs. You came down from upstairs and were expressing your appreciation to everyone." This indicates that M wants the therapist to be close to her as a family. The girl using drugs represented the lost part of M who had numbed and avoided her true pain as much as possible with drugs. In response, not only she but also her inner parents and the therapist are grieving, and the therapist is expressing his gratitude to the attendants as M's relative. This expressed that M was facing the problem of termination of treatment and wanted to internalize the therapist who understood the dead part of her painful self. The therapist playing the piano represents M's desire to introject even the good aspect of the therapist which M is unaware of.

After 2 and a half years, when treatment was coming to an end due to the therapist's job relocation, M had the following dream: "You were a bus driver and your other patients and I were on the bus. You said that you would turn left but accidentally entered the left side road and stopped. There was a park. Your patients all got off the bus and went into a manhole. I asked you if everybody was all right but you said nothing. When I opened the cover there was nobody, everybody was dead." This dream expressed that M thought terminating treatment at this point was not right and that she was anxious and discontent that she might end up like all the other therapist's patients, that is, they would be cut off treatment in mid-course and abandoned in a drainage path and die. When the therapist interpreted as so, M answered that "It is true that I have a huge sense of loss because you are going away and sometimes feel worried that I might die. I am very discontent and unhappy why you are not staying here as you are now."

Furthermore, M reported the following dream: "I was lying on the couch in the treatment room. There was a hole in the wall. You said you wanted to talk to the women in the next room and passed through the hole. When I looked with jealousy, there was a baby sitting on the bed. You were cradling the baby in your arms. I thought the woman in the next room was me." This dream expressed that M was thinking that even after treatment was terminated, she wanted to follow the therapist into the other world and pretend the separation with the therapist would never happen, and would like to live in the therapist's world and make a family. Furthermore, the baby the therapist was holding also represented M herself. When the therapist gave her these interpretations, M indicated her strong complaints, "That is true enough but why are you leaving when you are aware of it?" and expressed her fierce discontent that it was painful and she could not stand that treatment was going to end. M gradually accepted the experience of separation by repeatedly experiencing the omnipotent world of redemption united with God, feeling strong sadness and loneliness or sometimes directing her rage towards the therapist.

Resultingly, treatment continued for 2 years and 6 months but had to be terminated due to the therapist's job relocation. The therapist had an impression that although M was able to address and solve many inner tasks, she still had not completely introjected the world where the therapist understood and supported her. In that meaning, it seems to be difficult to say that the therapist's therapeutic goal was fully achieved. On the other hand, her symptoms had clinically improved and she had returned to her previous fulltime job. She was doing well at work; she bought a new home and the relationship with her family had no particular problems anymore.

5. Considerations

The issue of the therapeutic mechanism in psychoanalysis is largely related to the issues of the therapeutic goal, therapeutic technique and the termination of treatment. There also exists a fundamental question: From which perspective does the therapist understand the patient's unconscious pathological mental world, what kind of state the pathological problem is in and how does the therapist understand it? This has a strong relationship with the fundamental mental theory and technical theory which the therapist stands on. This paper first introduced Freud's fundamental perspective and technical theory, therapeutic mechanism and purpose and then introduced the therapeutic mechanism and goal based on the modern Kleinian perspectives and techniques.

As seen in the case, what the therapist mainly conducted in the therapeutic course is centred on the understanding of the unconscious meaning of the patient's expressions of free association. They were proceeded with, for example, splitting and projective identification, symbolic process and displacement. The fundamental of treatment techniques is to keep on giving interpretations with understandable words for the patient on the basis that the therapist understands the world of unconscious object relations related to the inner phantasy or the state of activities of the defensive world through the various contents expressed by the patient's free-associations and acting-outs. This part consists of the world of the conflictive pathological object relation filled with anxiety, which has been split-off from the patient's conscious world. The therapeutic relation is a relationship of container/contained. Through this, the patient works through to restore his/her split-off world into his/her self. As for the therapeutic process, the patient needs to have an experience in the former half where he/she is fully understood by the therapist. In the latter half, the centre of the process becomes the patient's introjection of the ability to understand his/her own problem from the therapist. The goal for the patient after the termination of treatment is to be able to take up his/her own unconscious conflictive tasks and understand and come up with a way to handle them with his/her own thought.

In the treatment of the above case, it seems that the patient was able to quite sufficiently have an experience where the therapist gave her interpretations of his understandings and she thought she was understood. However, there is a possibility that the patient experienced that she was a little rushed to separation in the latter half. Even so, since the patient reported many dreams that promoted self-understanding and had actually come to be able to understand those meanings well, it seems that she had considerably introjected the therapist's ability to think and understand. The criteria for the termination of treatment are: the patient becomes able to be aware of his/her conflict, address the problem, understand it on his/her own, think and find a solution to it, that is, to be able to acquire self-understanding with autonomy. Elimination of the conflicts is by no means the therapeutic goal or the criterion to evaluate the therapeutic efficacy.

References

(1) Bion, Wilfred Ruprecht. 1962. *Learning from experience*. London: Heinemann.

(2) Freud, Sigmund. 1914. "Remembering, repeating and working through", In *Standard Edition*, Vol. 12. London: Hogarth Press.

(3) Freud, Sigmund. 1917. "Mourning and Melancholia". In *Standard Edition*, Vol. 14. London: Hogarth Press.

(4) Freud, Sigmund. 1933. "New Introductory Lectures on Psychoanalysis". In *Standard Edition*, Vol. 22. London: Hogarth Press.

(5) Freud, Sigmund. 1937: "Analysis Terminable and Interminable". In *Standard Edition*, Vol.23. London: Hogarth Press.

(6) Hinshelwood, Robert Douglas. 1989: *A Dictionary of Kleinian Thought*. London: Free Association Books.

(7) Klein, Melanie. 1940/1975: "Mourning and its Relation to Manic-Depressive States". In *The writings of Melanie Klein*, Vol. 1. London: Hogarth Press.

(8) Klein, Melanie. 1946/1975. "Notes on Some Schizoid Mechanisms". In *The Writings of Melanie Klein*, Vol. 3. London: Hogarth Press.

(9) Money-Kyrle, Roger. 1971/1978. "The Aim of Psycho-Analysis". In *The Collected Papers of Roger Money-Kyrle*. Perthshire: Clunie Press.

(10) Rosenfeld, Herbert. 1964. "On the Psychopathology of Narcissism: A Clinical Approach". In *Psychotic States*. London: Hogarth Press.

(11) Rosenfeld, Herbert. 1971: "A Clinical Approach to the Psychoanalytic Theory of the Life and Death Instincts: An Investigation into the Aggressive Aspects of Narcissism". *International Journal of Psychoanalysis*, vol. 52: 169-178.

(12) Sandler, Joseph, and Dreher, Anna. 1996. *What Do Psychoanalysis Want?: The Problem of Aims in Psychoanalytic Therapy*. London: Routledge.

(13) Steiner, John. 1989. "The Aim of Psychoanalysis". *Psychoanalytical Psychotherapy*, Vol. 4: 109-120.

(14) Steiner, John. 1990. "Pathological Organization as Obstacles to Mourning: The Role of Unbearable Guilt" *International Journal of Psychoanalysis*, Vol. 71: 87-94.

(15) Steiner, John. 1993: *Psychic Retreats: Pathological Organizations of the Personality in Psychotic, Neurotic and Borderline Patients*. London & New York: Routledge.

(16) Steiner, John. 1996. "The Aim of Psychoanalysis in Theory and in Practice", *International Journal of Psychoanalysis*, Vol. 77: 1073-1083.

[2004. *The Japanese Journal of Psycho-analysis*, Vol. 48, No. 3]

CHAPTER 12

DYNAMICS OF INTERPRETING TRANSFERENCES

1. Introduction

Transference interpretation is one of the most important tasks of psychoanalysis and its theme is a central matter nearly equal to discussing psychoanalysis itself. Here I would like to describe the historical tasks and development of transference, the diversification of interpretation and the fundamental viewpoint for considering the meaning of transference interpretation contained in it. Furthermore, I would like to describe the characteristics of my basis, that is, emphasis on the understanding of unconscious transference in the object relation theory and emphasis on transference interpretation in "here-and-now".

2. Transition and meaning of the concept of transference

(1) S. Freud's study

J. Breuer treated Anna O from 1881 to 1882. It was when the phenomenon where the patient had a passionate romantic feeling for Breuer was observed that Freud knew about the phenomenon of transference love for the first time. Anna O's feeling made Breuer terminate therapy himself. Freud took a strong interest in this phenomenon and tried to see it scientifically considering it important for solving the pathology of hysteria. Additionally, Freud himself encountered the phenomenon of transference love during a hypnotic therapy with his own patient and focused on the universality and the importance of this phenomenon. However, Freud at that time did not consider that such transference love was important in therapy itself. Rather, he considered it as something that interfered with treatment.

It was in the Dora case (4) that Freud clearly featured the problem of transference. In this discontinued case, Freud revealed that there was the problem of Dora's ambivalent negative and positive transferences towards Freud in the background. However, Freud at that time still considered such transferences should be abandoned immediately because they would interfere with the therapy.

Later on, Freud began to think that the transference phenomenon was universal and, although it disturbs therapy, tracing the origin of it would become the key to treatment. Then, he began to consider that, along with the discovery of Oedipus complex, such infantile parents imago, especially the father imago, was transferred to the therapist. As he described in the case of Rat Man, he began to consider that solving the father transference was the key of therapy. However, Freud's handling of transferences was limited just to the world of conscious transferences, by re-construction and developmental interpretation.

Freud used concepts such as transference love, positive transference, negative transference, father transference, super-ego transference and transference neurosis to express the individual characteristics of the transference phenomena. These concepts are generally used even now.

(2) Development of the concept of transference by M. Klein

a Psychoanalysis for children (1932)

The new perspective of psychoanalysis began to develop from Klein's early analysis. Klein began to conduct psychoanalysis for very little children under 3 years old. It was called play therapy, which was performed with a technique where the meaning of the children's play was understood and interpreted. The fundamental method Klein adopted then was an application of the method of Freud's dream interpretation. In other words, Klein equated expressions of the children's play to manifest dreams and called what corresponded to the background latent dreams as unconscious phantasy. Thus, what is expressed through the children's play with processes such as condensation, symbolism and displacement is the world of unconscious phantasy, which is active in the then current unconsciousness. The fundamental technical perspective of "here-and- now" started here.

Furthermore, according to Klein, the children's world of unconscious phantasy is a projection of their 0-year-old internal world, which is filled with part-object-relational sadism with their parents. For little children, it is a reflection of the very recent world of experience with their parents. It internalizes the conflictive object relation with their parents, which is still currently ongoing at home.

Klein discovered that some of such internalized primitive experiences with their parents and the strong anxieties related to them are transferred to the therapist. She then reached to the conclusion that it was therapeutically important to interpret them with words that are understandable to children.

In this way, Klein gradually revealed the characteristics of the children's unconsciousness in child psychoanalysis. She considered that the world of children's unconsciousness was centred on persecutory anxiety filled with fear of aggression and retaliation based on sadism. She also considers that it is a world where part object relations and whole object relations are intricate where primitive defence systems including splitting, projection, introjection, denial, and omnipotence are active. Such worlds of anxiety and internal object relations are often expressed in children's play and the therapist's role is to understand them well and interpret them with words that children can understand.

b Psychoanalysis of adults

In the 1930's, Klein began to apply her experiences of treating children to treatment of adult manic-depressive disease and paranoia. In the treatment for Hans [(5)], Freud thought that little children, who do not have a sufficient language ability, are not subjects for psychoanalysis. Actually, the Hans's case was a case of guidance for the father.

Through the experiences of children's play therapy, Klein was struck with wonder that children's play expressed the rich inner world and came to assert that children's play was equivalent to adults' verbal free-association. From such perspective, she became to understand unconsciousness in play and came to think that psychoanalytic therapy could be conducted for very little children aged 2 to 3.

In addition, as Klein accumulated experiences of treating adults, she challenged the then common sense of psychoanalysis. She reversed the above-mentioned proposition and began to advocate that the content of adults' free-association was equivalent to children's play. She began to think that the content of the adults' associations was play and an indirect expression of the currently active unconscious phantasy. She also thought that the adults' verbal expressions were a poorer method for expression.

Put simply, Klein considered that the unconscious phantasy even during wakefulness is expressed in a distorted way such by condensation, displacement, or symbolism through adults' associations and acting-outs as in dreams. Klein explained that these actions, as she revealed in children's research, were functions of the primitive defence systems including projection, projective identification, denial, and omnipotence. She then discovered that the activity of the unconscious object relation in 0-year-olds, which she found in children's psychoanalysis, was expressed also in adults. More specifically, through her treatment experiences of manic-depressive disease and schizophrenia, Klein focused on the disposition of a 0-year-old in adult patients and began to emphasize the importance of the depressive position (6-month disposition) and the paranoid-schizoid position (3-month disposition). Furthermore, she thought that the origin of transference existed in these two positions.

She began to pay attention to the state of inner object relations, primitive defence systems, annihilation anxiety, persecutory anxiety, and depressive anxiety in these positions. She then began to emphasize that they are the components of unconscious phantasy and are greatly related to the transference to the therapist.

c Attention to unconscious transference

Klein had already focused on unconscious transference in children' play therapy. She considered that the children's unconsciousness was near the consciousness and clearly expressed, like open-cut mining, the object relation developed with the current fosterer through play.

Similarly, Klein created a path to understand the activity of the background unconscious phantasies through the associations of adult patients and further deepened her attention to unconscious transferences. The expressions of adults' verbal free-associations are poorer than those of children's play so the expression of the unconscious phantasy becomes distorted and ambiguous because of various defence mechanisms. That is, in the background of the content of adults' free-associations, which is equated to conscious dreams, unconscious phantasies are expressed while being influenced by various defence mechanisms. It is in quite a disguised state where the current therapeutic relation with the therapist, the transference relation, is unconsciously displayed, although it is not as easy to understand as children's play. This perspective is essentially associated to the clinical technique of "here-and-now" as state above.

Klein states that correspondence is often therapeutically too late when phenomena such as conscious transferences have appeared and says that it is therapeutically extremely important to understand, grasp, and interpret the unconscious transferences that have been evolving before them. This is a representative characteristic of Klein's technique.

Here lies a big question of how to understand the transference phenomena in clinical practice. It is related to the fundamental theoretical perspective and techniques of each group. Understanding of transference and the way to interpret the transferences in clinical practice largely differ among groups depending on where the origin of transference is placed, which developmental stage and aspect are focused on in the transference phenomena, and whether it is the conscious transference or the unconscious transference that is mainly seen, and other approaches.

d Kleinian understanding and interpretation of unconscious transferences

The Kleinian way to understand unconscious phantasy is to try to see its activities by reading between the lines of the content of associations and the subtle expressions of acting-ins and acting-outs. To do so, it is necessary to make clear the whole activity situation of the inner object relation at first. Then the therapist will understand phenomena such as unconscious transferences, unconscious defences, and unconscious inner anxieties. Transference cannot be interpreted without these understandings.

Technically, effort will be exercised to grasp the state of unconscious activity at the site of clinical practice through subtle materials of associations and acting-outs to understand the unconscious phantasies.

There are two processes for interpretation: first, it is the process of understanding such unconscious activities and second, it is the process of delivering the contents of the understandings to the patient through verbalization. Obviously, if the former interpretation, that is the understandings of the dynamics, is not correct, the verbalized interpretations will be irrelevant. Traditionally, it is said that interpretations include resistance interpretations, defence interpretations, transference interpretations, developmental interpretations, and interpretations of inner anxiety. Among them, transference interpretation has been considered the most important. It has been explored in clinical practice with trial and error as empirical science.

In the case of Kleinians, the centre of treatment is to find and interpret the unconscious transference in the activities of unconscious phantasies that are currently occurring at the site of therapy. This is considered as mutative interpretation, which is important as "here-and-now" intervention. However, in actual clinical practice, the other interpretations are also important. It is considered that an approach where the therapist appropriately allocates interpretations of outside-therapy transferences, developmental interpretations (reconstruction), and other interpretations and converges them to transference interpretations is appropriate.

3. Case presentation

(1) Case patient

The patient is a single Japanese woman N in her late 20s. She was an aspiring stage actor. Her main complaints were obsessive ideas, which had continued for about 20 years, compulsive act, chronic depressive state, general malaise, and severe constipation. The sudden death of the patient's father when she was young triggered the onset. She has a brother who is emotionally unstable, does not have a job and suffers from social self-identity disturbance. Her mother remarried six months after the death of the patient's father. Her new partner also lost his wife to a disease and had two daughters around the same age as N. N's mother was self-centred and dominating. N was dependent on her mother and called her everyday even though she lived far away. After N's mother remarried when N was a young girl, N's mother went alone to a faraway vocational school for a year so N lived apart from her mother with her stepfather's family. Although the above-mentioned neurological symptoms had continued since her childhood and slightly worsened in her adolescence; she somehow managed to do her academic work. N had a special strong interest in literature. Her symptoms including endless rechecking worsened because of various frictions of human relationships, so she came to the therapist for consultation. Treatment was conducted 3 times a week using a couch for psychoanalytic psychotherapy.

(2) Therapeutic course

A number of sessions during the first six months from the start of therapy are described here.

During the number of sessions after the therapist's summer vacation, the atmosphere was generally negative and pessimistic and the content of the conversation was mainly gloomy. N had broken up with her boyfriend B just before the vacation and was confused. N was dependent on her mother; however, her mother had gone to a resort spot leaving N alone. Furthermore, N was upset because her house owner had told her to leave her boarding house. Thereafter, she got back together with her boyfriend B but their relation had become more distant than before. B tried to have violent sex with N and she felt she was being exploited.

N emphasized an extremely pessimistic world saying, "I want to laugh when I am unhappy. I just become confused and painful when I come here." I, the therapist, felt quite painful and strongly experienced a sense where there was no exit when being told these complaints and denials. This expresses the patient's world of expectation, disappointment, complaint, and aggression towards the object. In this world, she did not try to accept the value of the therapy which provided a positive experience for her and she expressed her emotions such as anger, revenge, intense feeling of guilt and fear. This was contrary to before the vacation when N was going well with B and a proactive self-understanding was making progress.

(3) Sessions

I would like to report a number of sessions in the 3rd week after the vacation in details and introduce the state of the unconscious phantasies and the actual of the transference interpretation.

a The Zth session

N spoke in a rather abrupt manner on a chair without using the couch. She said she had a daydream. N had often had daydreams from her childhood. Recently, B recommended N to write a scenario. When the therapist asked about the daydream, N said, "It was about B. There was a man D who said he could write a scenario. B had just started a project for a new play. However, I was heavily injured and almost had myself killed. B came to see me and discontinued the project. Mother was near me and was very flustered. Also, my friend's boyfriend came but I ignored him."

The therapist interpreted the daydream to N as follows: "You are crying over your inability and are envious about B's success. When the surrounding people leave you and make light of you without appreciating you, you think that if you get heavily injured, B, your mother and all your friends would run to you risking everything for you. And you want to confirm that you are the most important existence. You feel that you cannot tell your various confusing experiences about the vacation as you want to in therapy and it seems that you want me, the therapist, to also run to you and support you."

Continuously, N told another daydream: N has a boss. He is attractive and more than 10 years older than her. N feels that the boss is like her father. The boss feels N is like his daughter. He sometimes lends N money. He joins the conversation on women's weeklies and talks casually with N. However, N added, "Actually, my boss is strict to me."

Furthermore, N said, "I am not creative today." N said that it was very important whether she was creative or not. This may be because she is sensitively concerned whether she is accepted by the therapist or not and the world of death lives together in her inner world.

Additionally, N told a story that a foreign Asian woman taught her a local word meaning "not being in the centre of your mind". N commented, "If I place myself in the centre, even if I said I didn't want to and refused to clean the basement, the cleaning lady would give me due respect and show a different reaction to me." N continued "It is important to be in the centre of myself when I am an actor. If I am in the centre, I can play well."

The therapist interpreted this as follows: "That woman is a foreigner. Saying that you are not in the centre of your mind probably means that you have lost your own spontaneous world. You feel that I am saying something like that to you. It seems that you are thinking that if you were in a spontaneous world, I would not treat you with little regard even if you said you didn't want to clean your mental basement."

Although N said "If I was in my spontaneous world, I could act truly," this is a rather conflicting story. This probably means that if she was in the centre of her self, she could also act the other roles very realistically, but if she were not, she would reveal her inefficiency.

N said "I do not think I am saying anything creative today. Can I smoke a cigarette?" Not being creative probably meant that she would unintentionally show her void and disturbed self.

The therapist interpreted this as follows: "You are worried that I would not accept you if you were not creative. You are anxious that if you do not show your firm side, other emotions that are more unstable like a child would come out. You are hurt deep down inside so you are asking me to help you. You want me to put everything aside and help you preferentially. Your daydreams say so."

However, N did not agree saying, "The daydreams are about B and my boss so they have nothing to do with therapy." This was N's usual reaction to express she did not agree with the therapist's interpretations. However, N's associations advanced and showed a new development, therefore the therapist did not think the interpretations were completely wrong.

N continuously gave associations: "All the machineries, the washing machine, the radio, etc. were not working well. B came to use the radio but the reception was bad. We could not hear the usual program using standard Japanese but heard a program using a dialect."

This was a very interesting association. The therapist sometimes spoke in not standard Japanese but in a dialect. I felt that a transference relation was actively moving at the site so I decided to give an interpretation on the spot for such a representative utterance.

I, the therapist interpreted, "I cannot the speak standard Japanese well. So, you find it difficult talking to me. You feel that I am insufficient for a therapist and I cannot understand what you are expressing or help you."

N answered, "It is just a coincidence. Why do you take it that way?" and denied my interpretation, as usual. I continued, "It is related to your anxiety about the difference of local cultures, whether you will be understood or not."

N opposed this and countered, "But this is just a coincidence. You are reacting too sensitively." Continuously, N said "Last night, I wondered if you thought I am intelligent. Because I talk too much about childish things. I want to be intelligent. I want to be intelligent to acquire independence." Being intelligent is what N appealed recently, which seems to express the aspect of the intellectual defence. The therapist interpreted as follows:

"Being intelligent is being an adult. Aren't you feeling that you will not be accepted by me if you show your childish feature?"

N looked irritated and insecure and said rapidly, "Isn't time over? I have nothing to say. I don't want to be here. Because if my baby mind comes out, I will not want to leave here. I want to be independent and intelligent. However, I am not behaving like an adult in practice. I cannot even move out of my boarding house."

The therapist interpreted, "You have an attachment for your boarding house and also for this room." N pleaded once again, "I do not think so. You will know if we change rooms."

I told her "Also, you rely on me too. When there is a vacation, you will be on shaky grounds," but N denied, "I do not think so. I come here to be intelligent. Even if my attachment comes to the surface, there are no solutions when I leave here so I do not want to rely on anyone."

N said, "Because you will leave me in the end, too. Everybody will die. It's not fair. You are too kind so I want you to be unkind sometimes." The therapist interpreted, "No one will help you when you have such experience of losing someone. I think it is something that you fear the most; you feel you are isolated and are exposed to a world where no one helps you." N left the consultation room with an anxious look.

b The Z+1th session

N began to take lectures and read books on psychoanalysis. N had a strong interest in the therapist's world, however on the other hand, it seemed that N, who tried to arm herself with intelligence, hated my action to try to look at the activity of her upset infantile world and her other worlds.

N said, "B does not try to take me out. I wonder why? At B's first stage, his parents and brothers were there. He left me alone and spoke with another female actor. He made me talk with his family and mother. I was very disappointed."

In such way, N indirectly expressed her ambivalence of dependence on the therapist in her associations. This was related to the fact that the therapist was going to take the following week off. I interpreted, "It is related to the next 2 cancelations. You are feeling that you are treated without consideration and are rejected because I do not try to take you to my personal world."

After N replied, "It has nothing to do with you. I am talking about B. I don't know anything about you," she gave an association, "When I am in this consultation room, I recall my room when I was a university student. I shared a room with my friend at university." She continued her association, "It is also similar to the room which I lived in with my older step-sister, my step-father's daughter, when my mother remarried." In such way, N developed her associations while always denying the therapist's intervention. This probably displays that the therapist's intervention was right.

The therapist said, "You do not know if I understand you but you seem to feel that I am close like a cohabiter and that you share something with me."

N subsequently talked about a baby. "When I was 13 years old, I baby-sat. The 10-month-old baby did not stop crying. He didn't stop even if I touched his penis. I did something I shouldn't have. I feel a sense of guilt. I might have hurt him."

She further talked about a man at her office: "I am troubled because he asks me to do many things without any explanation when there are no people around. He makes me associate with him for everything like playing games of bridge, doing personal matters and tax matters. I am angry about that. My boss doesn't explain anything so I am mad."

N gave an important association here. The baby who did not stop crying whom she was responsible for taking after expresses the baby part of the abandoned N. N tried to calm it down with sexual excitement but failed and felt a strong sense of guilt about that. The therapist who is going to take a vacation just forced the session cancellation on N and left her in a troubled situation without any explanation. It can be considered that N had a strong discontent and anger against such therapist. The therapist gave the following interpretation: "You are also mad when I do not answer your questions. I think you are talking about your baby mind being left alone because of my vacation. You feel you are rejected and are angry when you are left alone. Sexual excitement may be your only consolation."

N replied to this and said, "Sex with B has a big meaning." The therapist interpreted, "B refuses to deal with you and does not take you out. I will leave you alone because of my vacation. It seems that sexual excitement is the only consolation to calm down your loneliness and anger."

N said, "When my grandmother died when I was 16, I began to masturbate and became excited. I felt a strong sense of guilt about that. I thought that my dead grandmother might be looking down on me from somewhere. It was something that betrayed my ethnic moral."

c The Z+4th session

N cancelled the Z+3th session and in the following session she complained of depression and a headache. N had a dream about her aunt and then had the following dream: "I was walking on the street with my friends. There was an open-bar and young gang members were walking. A woman was spreading her legs and seducing men. There were bad gangs and I belonged to the worse group. The previous good group I belonged to was boring. I had a good time and went to a pool. I was sinking coffins with dead bodies into the pool. There was a beautiful lady and we masturbated together." In addition, N had another dream two days before: "I was at a theatre and someone said to me that I was ugly. I wanted to get out but I didn't know where the exit was. I asked someone and went out from the back of the stage. The place was Tokyo. Tokyo is the place where my friend C worked (C is rich and successful.). We were all having lunch at a large table. I didn't like that." The former dream has a theme regarding a manic defence for object loss and the latter dream is related to the theme of expectation, disappointment, and envy towards the therapist. When associations and dreams are evolving like this, it can be considered that the therapist's approach is approximately pertinent.

4. Basic techniques and understanding of unconscious transferences

Although the style of expression of the patient N is verbal expression in these sessions, the process of understanding the background unconscious phantasies is quite complicated. At the therapeutic site of Kleinian object relation theory, the following fundamental perspective of the therapist underlies in the process. Although it is difficult to grasp every flow of the fluid unconscious phantasies at the actual clinical site, the therapist's ability will be tested how much closer he/she can come to the centre of the dynamics of the partial movements.

The therapist should fundamentally maintain the state called "free floating attention" (S. Freud) and "no memory, no desire" (W. R. Bion) as much as possible and keep on holding a sensation for various information. All the materials expressed by the patient including free associations, acting-outs and counter-transferences are appearances of the activity of the unconscious phantasies at that moment (although it is only partial). It is expressed by phenomena such as displacement, symbolism, and condensation similar to dreams during sleep. In other words, it is expressed euphemistically by the action of the primitive defence systems such as splitting, projective identification and denial.

For the therapist, it is important to listen attentively to the free associations and pick up the meaning of them. While doing so, the therapist will grasp the state of the phenomena such as resistance, defence, transference, and central anxiety. They have been further discussed from the following perspectives. At the actual therapeutic site, the therapist makes effort to pay attention to all of these points.

The fundamental perspective of container/contained and reverie is something that focuses on the subjective relationship between the therapist and the patient, and is a relationship of comprehension or understanding (reverie) focused on projective identification and introjective identification and basic communication centred on counter-transference. On that foundation, therapists gather materials (verbal expressions, non-verbal expressions, acting-outs, acting-ins, counter-transferences, etc.) and grasp the meaning of unconscious phantasies such as unconscious motivations. Sorting is conducted there whether the therapist has appropriately selected facts based on his/her α-function, or whether the therapist has not given excessive meanings due to counter-transferences. Especially, attention is paid to counter-transferences. There are acting-outs based on not only the therapist's affective situation but also the therapist's subtle counter-transferences, which have been pointed out by concepts such as "nagging" by B. Joseph, and "collusion" by J. Steiner, which drive the therapist to subtle acting-outs. Furthermore, it becomes important to understand the world of object relations focused on persecutory anxiety (paranoid-schizoid position) and depressive anxiety (depressive position) based on the structural perspective of the part-self of the pathological organization (J. Steiner). In this paper, I have mainly presented the description of a case patient; therefore, those theoretical perspective are stated only briefly.

Such function of the therapist often becomes clear through not only the therapist's introspection, training, and clinical experience but also through experiences of supervision and opinions from a third party at study meetings. An important prerequisite for those who conduct psychoanalysis and psychoanalytical psychotherapy is to participate in study meetings for lifelong learning and to always avoid becoming isolated and maintain the stance where they can listen to opinions of a third party.

As for the significance of transference interpretation, as is well known, it is important that the patient becomes aware of the experiences he/she has with the therapist at the therapeutic site, as a site of psychic reality, through interpretation and that this becomes a self-mutative therapeutic experience. Even in outer reality descriptions or seemingly meaningless subtle conversations, the patient is definitely describing a part of his/her self which connects to the therapist and the relationship through the unconscious motivation that selected the theme and the patient's own projective identifications. The important therapeutic task for the therapist is to reveal the unconscious transference with a continuous attitude to seek the transference relationship which is always latent in the background.

5. Conclusion

This paper has introduced a historical consideration on transference interpretation centring on Freud. Furthermore, it has focused on the historical development of Kleinian transference understanding from children's play therapy to the treatment of adult psychosis and has shown its revolutionary nature. A relatively detailed clinical course was presented, too. Although many theoretical developments regarding these clinical processes can be seen, only an overview has been introduced due to space limitations.

References

(1) Bion, Wilfred Ruprecht. 1963. *Elements of Psychoanalysis*. London: Heinemann.

(2) Bion, Wilfred Ruprecht. 1970. *Attention and Interpretation*. London: Tavistock Publications.

(3) Britton, Ron. 1989. *Belief and Imagination*. London: Routledge.

(4) Freud, Sigmund. 1905. "Fragment of an analysis of a case of hysteria". In *Standard Edition*, Vol. 7. London: Hogarth Press.

(5) Freud, Sigmund. 1909. "Analysis of a Phobia in a Five-Year-Old Boy". In *Standard Edition*, Vol. 10. London: Hogarth Press.

(6) Freud, Sigmund. 1923. "The Ego and the Id". In *Standard Edition*, Vol. 19. London: Hogarth Press.

(7) Heimann, Paula. 1950. "On Counter-Transference". *International Journal of Psychoanalysis*, Vol. 31: 81-84.

(8) Hinshelwood, Robert Douglas. 1989. *A dictionary of Kleinian Thought*. London: Free Association Books.

(9) Joseph, Betty. 1989. *Psychic Equilibrium and Psychic Change*. London: Routledge.

(10) Klein, Melanie. 1932/1975. "Psychoanalysis of Children". In *The Writings of Melanie Klein*, Vol. 2. London: Hogarth Press.

(11) Klein, Melanie. 1952/1975. "On the Origin of Transference". In *The Writings of Melanie Klein*, Vol. 3, London: Hogarth Press.

(12) Racker, Heinrich. 1968. *Transference and Countertransference*. London: Hogarth Press.

(13) Rosenfeld, Herbert. 1983. "Primitive Object Relations and Mechanisms". *International Journal of Psychoanalysis*, Vol. 64: 261-267.

(14) Segal, Hanna. 1981. *The Work of Hanna Segal: A Kleinian Approach to Clinical Practice*. New York: Jason & Aronson.

(15) Spillius, Elizabeth Both. ed. 1988. *Melanie Klein Today*, Vol.1, Vol.2. London: Routledge.
(16) Steiner, John. 1993. *Psychic Retreats*. London: Routledge.

[2008. *The Japanese Journal of Psycho-analysis*, Vol. 52, No. 3.]

CHAPTER 13

A-T SPLIT AND STRUCTURAL THEORY

1. Introduction

The clinical setting of A-T split began to be advocated in clinical studies of borderline cases. "A" stands for the Administrator and "T" stands for the Therapist, respectively. The A-T split is a procedure where separate clinicians such as doctors, psychologists, social workers, and public health nurses are responsible for each role in the treatment of patients with pathological personalities such as borderline patients who are subject to psychoanalytic psychotherapy. A-T split is a therapeutic structure that was first adopted at Menninger Clinic for inpatient treatment of borderline patients, and it is now applied also to outpatient treatment and other treatments. This setting was advocated mainly because it was felt that a cooperative staff relationship was necessary when treating patients with borderline personality disorder who show acting-out such as self-injurious behaviour, overdosing, or suicide attempts, and unstable emotional instability in interpersonal relationships. It is a system in which the administrator is in charge of overall management, and the therapist concentrates on psychoanalytic psychotherapy. The role of the administrator ranges from giving necessary advice, instructions, and medications, corresponding to acting-out, arranging hospitalizations, contacting emergency doctors to having interviews with family members, and in the case of pubertal/adolescent patients, cooperating with schools and police. By undertaking all these roles, the administrator aims to support the basic structure of psychoanalytical psychotherapy and let the psychotherapist focus on psychoanalytic psychotherapy.

It has been empirically confirmed that such a setting where the administrator and the therapist are different doctors works most effectively in patients with severe self-injurious behaviour or self-destructive acting-out, who are subject to psychoanalytical psychotherapy.

In fact, in the psychoanalytical psychotherapy research group the author belongs to, the A-T split method is applied to most patients who are undergoing psychotherapy and the member doctors mutually take charge of the patients as the administrator or the therapist.

The A-T split is actually a part of an overall therapeutic structure setting. If there is no overall structural understanding, even when A-T split is adopted superficially, it will not work therapeutically. In addition, doctors who play the role of the administrator often have difficulty in making appropriate decisions and approaching patients and their families if they do not have experience in psychoanalytic psychotherapy. However, even in such cases, they can give much support if they have an affinity to psychoanalytic psychotherapy. If the administrator is uncomfortable with psychoanalytical psychotherapy, when the patient's acting-out becomes more aggressive or a negative therapeutic response occurs during the course of treatment, the administrator may assert that it is because the psychotherapist is not handling it well, or may begin to criticize due to a misunderstanding that psychoanalytic psychotherapy not only has no therapeutic effect, but also exacerbates the patient's conditions.

Understanding of the background overall structure theory is essential for the actual clinical significance of A-T split.

The therapeutic structure theory was advocated by Dr. Keigo Okonogi in Japan. It is the most basic of basic viewpoint when conducting psychoanalytic psychotherapy and A-T split is also implemented based on that concept. Dynamic developmental diagnosis is performed for all cases to which psychoanalytic psychotherapy may be applicable. When the patient is considered eligible for psychoanalytic psychotherapy, then it is decided which therapeutic structure is to be used for treatment.

2. Dynamic Developmental Diagnosis and A-T Split

Dynamic developmental diagnosis is an organizational diagnosis performed in patients considered to be applicable to psychoanalytical psychotherapy such as patients with personality disorder. This diagnostic process can also be regarded as an important element of the therapeutic structure. This is because, based on the result of this diagnosis, it is determined whether psychoanalytical psychotherapy should be adopted or not, and when the patient is eligible for psychoanalytic psychotherapy, the location and frequency of treatment, selection of therapist, necessity of A-T split and other details will be considered. In psychiatric clinical practice in countries where human resources are abundant like European countries, the interviewer of dynamic developmental diagnosis, the administrator and the therapist are often different doctors or medical staff. This may be difficult depending on the circumstances of each country, region, or facility.

The actual dynamic developmental diagnosis is performed as follows. It is a structurally formalized diagnosis.

(1) A structural dynamic developmental diagnostic interview

After undergoing a general psychiatric diagnosis, when the patients are diagnosed with disorders such as personality disorder, a structural dynamic developmental diagnostic interview is conducted for those who may be eligible for psychoanalytical psychotherapy. Specifically, one session of 45 to 50 minutes is performed four times. In that process, necessary information will be collected to clarify details including the patient's pathology and treatment motivations, and it will be judged whether psychoanalytic psychotherapy can be applied or not.

(2) Check items for dynamic developmental diagnosis

The actual diagnostic interviews are not conducted in an interrogational form, but will be carried out thoroughly based on the patient's free self-expressions. The diagnostic interviewer has a list of items of the necessary information in the background, and interposes questions as necessary while the patient expresses him/herself freely. The list of check items that the diagnostic interviewer has in the background include the followings:

1) Situation of onset: It is often related to a conflicting situation in which the patient's defence mechanism breaks down.
2) Patient's living status from infancy to the present: especially peer experience during adolescence, etc.
3) Characteristics of current interpersonal relationships
4) Family description: parents' upbringing, experience of deprivation within the family from the time of grandparents, whether the patient has traumatic experience or not, etc.
5) Emotional state at the interview site, state of early transference
6) Dream, earliest memory, etc.

In addition to the above items, it is necessary to make a differential diagnosis of layered-clothes syndrome. The patients with layered-clothes syndrome are patients who clinically show a state of personality disorder or neurotic disorder but actually have an extremely mild pervasive developmental disorder in the background. In most of the patients with layered-clothes syndrome, psychoanalytic psychotherapy, which promotes self-understanding to understand the unconscious world, is not applicable. The combination of a supportive educational approach and drug therapy is therapeutically the most effective for them. During the dynamic diagnostic interview, items to distinguish this layered-clothes syndrome will also be checked. Furthermore, since it is necessary to confirm features such as the bias of cognitive function by psychological tests, the dynamic diagnostic interview will structurally take 6 hours in total including the time for the WEIS and Rorschach tests.

If this dynamic developmental diagnosis interview is not conducted firmly, it becomes hard to judge how to conduct a structural approach even to the patients who are considered eligible for psychoanalytic psychotherapy. Then, it becomes difficult to determine whether A-T split should be adopted or not, and consider what kind of problems may occur if the A-T split is not adopted.

(3) Judgement of dynamic development diagnosis and A-T split

In the 4th session of the dynamic developmental diagnostic interviews, the diagnostic interviewer needs to give the patient the results of the judgment and a clear opinion on what kind of treatment is appropriate for him/her. When the interviewer considers that psychoanalytic psychotherapy is appropriate, he/she will state so accordingly. Then, the interviewer needs to explain the points including what kind of structure the treatment will be conducted in, and confirm whether the patient has a motivation to receive treatment. At that time, the interviewer also needs to explain the A-T split procedure.

When the results of the dynamic developmental diagnostic session and psychological tests come out, the overall judgement is made while basically giving a consideration on the followings:

1) The therapeutic motivation
2) The trigger for onset: The patient often has a conflicting experience that breaks the defence mechanism which the patient had worn.
3) Painful experiences, conflict experiences: What were the painful and traumatic experiences, which were difficult to handle in life history for the patient, like?
4) Defence mechanism: How has the patient dealt with such painful and traumatic experiences?
5) Whether the patient shows self-destructive acting-out or not
6) How the patient expresses the inner world, and how he/she develops pathological object relations of interpersonal relations surrounding him/her through current interpersonal relations, dreams, and earliest memory, etc.
7) What kind of understanding the patient shows when the diagnostic interviewer explains the final results and tells him/her that

psychoanalytic psychotherapy is appropriate
8) What kind of transference relationship is considered to develop when treatment is started?

By examining the above matters in detail, the therapeutic structure will be determined concretely when psychoanalytical psychotherapy is to be performed. In other words, details will be considered, including the choice of the therapist, the treatment frequency, the choice of face-to-face or lying-down method, A-T split, drug administration, explanation to the family, possibility of hospitalization, possibility of self-destructive behaviour such as self-injurious behaviour and suicide attempt, and necessity of a network to correspond in such cases, and necessary points will be discussed with the patient and family. The administrator plays an important role here.

3. The therapeutic structure of psychoanalytical psychotherapy

As described above, the therapeutic structure is determined according to the pathology and realistic conditions of the patient. In the background, there is an organizational viewpoint based on the therapeutic structure. According to the therapeutic structure theory, the basic problems are considered from the following viewpoints.

(1) External therapeutic structure

This is a therapeutic structure setting in terms of time and space. Psychoanalytical therapy is a treatment method using free-association in a lying-down method with no duration limit, which is conducted for 45 to 50 minutes 4 to 5 times a week. This structural setting is the basis of psychoanalytic therapy and psychoanalytic psychotherapy. On the other hand, one session is also conducted for 45 to 50 minutes in psychoanalytic psychotherapy, but the frequency is 1 to 3 times a week in a face-to-face method or a lying-down method. Free association is used for conversation. Furthermore, in order to maintain the therapeutic structure, it is necessary to consider the physical structure and organization of the entire facility.

(2) Structure of staff deployment and A-T split

It is necessary to specifically determine the staff deployment based on not only the above-mentioned basic external structure but also the patient's pathology. That is, if self-destructive acting-out of patients with moderate or severer diseases such as personality disorder is anticipated, or if there is a possibility that problems including exacerbation of symptoms or emotional instability become exposed, not only psychotherapy, but also drug therapy, hospital treatment, cooperation with the emergency department, and cooperation with family members, school and police personnel and other surrounding people become important peripheral therapeutic structures. At this point, the main subject of A-T split arises. The psychotherapist needs to select the options for patients with such pathology, taking into consideration factors such as experience, sex, and age. On the other hand, the administrator needs to make a preliminary prediction at the time of the dynamic diagnostic interview on to what extent the basic structure should be maintained and management be conducted. In fact, when applying psychoanalysis or psychoanalytic psychotherapy to patients with various personality disorders who visit the outpatient department of psychiatry, it is often necessary to maintain the overall therapeutic structure through extensive structuralization and management by the administrator. Furthermore, it becomes an important point in the course of treatment that the administrator understands his/her position and role well in the therapeutic structure centred on psychoanalytic psychotherapy, and makes appropriate judgments and conducts appropriate management.

(3) Maintenance of the therapist-patient relationship

It is important for the administrator to understand the importance of constructing and maintaining the overall therapeutic structure based on A-T split. The overall therapeutic structure includes basic understanding of the facility and staff, and setting and maintenance of the support system and physical therapeutic structure. It is not until the administrator understands this importance well that the psychoanalytical psychotherapist can have a therapeutic encounter with the patient in a fixed interview room. Under these fixed conditions of time and space, the same therapist keeps a constant neutral and therapeutic attitude based on attentive listening and acceptance to understand the unconscious world and talk with the patient. This is the basic therapeutic structure.

In the actual treatment for personality disorder, the psychoanalytical psychotherapist (therapist) can devote him/herself to a dyadic psychotherapy with the patient at considerable ease, because the administrator conducts management to maintain the external therapeutic structure. Under such conditions, the therapist can maintain the most appropriate conditions to interact with the deep world of the patient. Under a constant structure, the inner world of the patient is projected onto the therapist, administrator, and the entire therapeutic structure. Since the structure is maintained constant, it becomes easy to grasp the clinical course including transferences and counter-transferences.

The therapist keeps on taking a neutral and "free-floating attitude", retains his/her unconscious sensitivity and can make full use of his/her emotions and thoughts, and can find and listen attentively to the expressions of unconscious fragments of the patient's associations. It becomes easy for the therapist to continuously retain the specific therapeutic attitude in such a therapeutic structure environment. The therapeutic mindset of the therapist is prone to fall into a state which is difficult to retain under an unstable structure such as general clinical practice, however, it becomes possible to preserve it under such a therapeutic structure.

On the other hand, it becomes very important for the administrator to maintain the surrounding physical therapeutic environment and the major structure, and to keep approaching various external structural problems through management. This is just like supporting child-rearing mothers. The husband, grandparents, the other family members, and surrounding people, try to make long-term adjustments for the children's growth by keeping the child-raising environment as steady as possible without breaking the delicate world of the mother-child relationship in order to make the state of the mother, who is absorbed in raising infants, as stable as possible.

4. Meanings of therapeutic structure and A-T split from the patients' viewpoint

After the time and space are set and the therapist and administrator are determined, psychoanalytical psychotherapy starts. The question is: "What kind of subjective and therapeutic experience will the patient have?"

The administrator organizationally conducts detailed diagnostic interviews, decides whether psychoanalytic psychotherapy is applicable or not based on that diagnosis, and allocates peripheral therapeutic structures and the therapist group. For the patient, this process is an experience which clearly presents the treatment policy and provides a great sense of safety and security. The state where the administrator and the therapist cooperate while playing their respective roles in A-T split strengthens the sense of trust and sense of safety, and the state where they attempt together to overcome various crises which happen in the therapeutic process brings about a stable sense of trust to the patient.

Of course, most patients have conflicting images of parents in their life history. Patients with severe personality disorder who have a destructive combined parent image tend to possess a strong suspicion and a sense of being excluded as transferences towards such a couple of the therapist and the administrator, who unitedly try to stretch out a helping hand to the patient. Additionally, in many cases, the patients develop a negative primitive transference relationship by projectively identifying with the destructive parents who scheme an aggressive plot against the patient in the background. The therapist needs to pay attention not only to such patient's transference to the therapist-administrator couple but also to the patient's subjective experience about the facility and the overall structure where other staff exist.

The patient continues to express his/her own world to the same therapist who takes the same attitude, and the therapist responds from a neutral, stable, and specific perspective, in the same space, that is, the interview room, for a certain amount of sufficient time. This experience is an experience which greatly vibrates the inside of the patient's mind. It can have a non-invasive and therapeutic impact on the pathological inner world. Such setting provides a therapeutic experience that reaches the depths which is most regulated by and important to the human mind. It is a specifically set space that differs from everyday space and interpersonal relationships. Even if the patient's primitive and unique world develops, the setting provides conditions of space and relationship with people, where the patient himself/herself can prevent diffusion and confusion of his/her emotions by means of the structure. Under those conditions, the patient touches his/her pathological parts and regressive parts and experiences that he/she can express them with a considerable sense of safety. The experience of a regular and repetitive therapeutic space also provides the patient with the therapist's object constancy and stability. It is a structural therapeutic environment where the patient can gradually come in touch with the condition of his/her depth and actually feel the existence of the therapist who can approach that world in a neutral and non-invasive manner. In such an environment, the patient feels guaranteed that he/she can express him/herself freely and expresses a primitive and pathological world that cannot be touched in everyday interpersonal relationships. Thus, the patient can develop self-understanding in cooperation with the therapist.

5. Case Report

I will describe a case here. Based on my experience as an administrator, I would like to introduce the role that management played in the course of treatment. (Information has been omitted or revised except for the essential parts regarding the purpose.)

Patient

The patient is Mr. B, a male patient in his twenties. His background included digestive dysfunction, self-injurious behaviour, repeated suicide attempts such as overdosing and jumping-off, and borderline personality disorder.

Family

His mother was a vicious drinker and repeatedly wasted money on gambling, and his father was emotionally unstable and strict. He had been a stern person since the patient's childhood, and Mr. B had always been afraid of him. His mother was at the mercy of his father and has been masochistically and passively living with him. She had repeatedly been in depressed states and had committed suicide. Mr. B's older brother gave up on the family early and has moved away from them.

Course of the medical consultation

Mr. B developed symptoms including anxiety and gastrointestinal disorders 6 years before the initial consultation due to trouble with his girlfriend. Since then, his symptoms waxed and waned, but on the other hand, Mr. B was a very hard-worker and a person with a strong super-ego. He obtained a professional qualification under extremely spatially and temporally harsh conditions. During this time, his emotions were unstable, and he repeatedly had anxious-depressive attacks and gastrointestinal disorders which were triggered by a trifle conflict in interpersonal relationships. Three years ago, he was admitted to the department of psychiatry because his condition worsened due to conflicts in interpersonal relationships and he suffered from emotional instability, difficulty in interpersonal relationships, and suicide attempts due to overdoses. After that, he frequently visited the emergency department with panic attack-like symptoms. Since then, he has been emotionally unstable and has repeated depressive states, jumping off and overdosing and has been in and out of hospital.

Mr. B was recommended psychoanalytic psychotherapy by his former doctor and was referred to me. Dynamic developmental diagnoses were conducted four times, and thereafter, psychoanalytic psychotherapy was introduced and A-T split was adopted. Here, I would like to outline the course of treatment from the perspective of an administrator and present the importance of A-T split.

Treatment course and function of the administrator

Mr. B cancelled sessions many times even after psychotherapy started. He continued to enjoy his nightlife, have digestive disorders and be at strife with his parents, and repeated hospitalization because of self-injurious behaviour and overdosing. He would resume psychotherapy after discharge, however, he cancelled sessions every other week and stayed at his friends' house to escape from his family who kept complaining to the patient, or went out late at night and returned home early in the morning.

Regarding hospitalization and treatment, mainly for worsening of symptoms and self-injurious behaviour, Mr. B's parents often asked for consultations with the administrator. They complained that they thought it was economically wasteful as there was no change, and relentlessly demanded explanations for the prospect of treatment and the necessity of hospitalization. Every time, the administrator needed to repeatedly give explanations such that inpatient treatment would be required if overdoses were repeated or gastrointestinal disorders were severe, and immediate results could not be obtained because psychotherapy required a long time. The patient participated in only about a total of a dozen psychotherapy sessions in the first year of psychotherapy since he repeated overdose emergency visits and hospitalization for gastrointestinal disorders several times. The administrator had to keep in close contact with the hospital doctor and be involved in arranging hospitalizations and discharges while supporting Mr. B who indicated his intention to receive therapy although he kept on cancelling sessions. It was a period when the administrator had to make many adjustments with Mr. B's family.

The administrator saw such a situation as the patient's negative initial transference in the introduction stage of psychoanalytic psychotherapy and as a representation of anxiety and confusion. Thus, the administrator adopted a policy to maintain the treatment time of psychotherapy as long as Mr. B was willing to continue psychotherapy, even if there were many cancellations. This was because the administrator considered that this introduction of psychotherapy was the last chance for Mr. B too, for 6 years had already passed from the onset of the disease, and he had previously dropped out of counselling a number of times, had made visits to many clinics and hospitals, and had repeated hospitalizations and discharges. In the meantime, Mr. B, who had been hospitalized for about a month several times, began to participate in psychotherapy regularly from the time he was hospitalized for 3 months in the first year of psychotherapy.

While discussing with the therapist, the administrator continued, under difficult circumstances, to secure psychotherapy sessions for Mr. B, deal with various acting outs and worsening of symptoms, and persuade the family who opposed hospitalization. This was probably the first time when Mr. B's feeling of trust towards the therapist and the administrator outweighed his distrust and anxiety. Mr. B began to appear for psychotherapy when he was about to be discharged, and after discharge, he began to come for therapy with almost no cancellations. Thereafter, gastrointestinal disorders and depression became stronger every few months, and he was repeatedly hospitalized and discharged for a relatively short period of time. However, the patient continued to attend psychotherapy during hospitalization except when his physical symptoms were extremely severe.

Mr. B's family still often complained to the administrator that it was a waste of money to hospitalize the patient who did not show improvement, but the administrator patiently explained to the family the necessity of hospitalization and the importance of psychotherapy each time. As the patient's condition tended to improve over time, his family no longer expressed their distrust against psychotherapy or complaints about hospitalization.

Since then, Mr. B has continued to participate in psychotherapy almost without any cancellations. Although his gastrointestinal disorders recurred every few months, and anxiety and illness were seen in association to the subject of treatment, his improved condition had been maintained for a relatively long period of time, and his condition was changing for the better in a wavelike manner. Basically, Mr. B progressed his self-understanding, and did not have any more previously seen overdoses or suicide attempts, and the amount of medication drastically decreased.

As shown above, in the case of a relatively severe personality disorder such as Mr. B, difficult problems including overdosing, self-injurious behaviour, and suicide attempts may repeatedly occur during the treatment introduction period, and the patient may repeat hospitalization and discharge. This means that there exists a group of patients who cannot regularly participate in psychotherapy from the beginning of treatment.

The administrator needs to concentrate on maintaining the treatment structure based on A-T split, by proactively responding to matters related to the outer frame of the treatment structure, such as medication, cooperation with hospital doctors, explanation to and adjustment with family members.

The administrator cannot function well without understanding the pathological characteristics of such patients and the importance of maintaining the therapeutic structure. In order to do so, it is desirable that the administrator forms a medical team him/herself and has therapeutic experience as a psychotherapist for patients with pathologies such as borderline personality disorder who repeat pathological acting outs.

6. Conclusion

A-T split has been practiced as an important element of the therapeutic structure mainly in psychoanalytic psychotherapy for patients with relatively severe personality disorders. It is built on the background basic therapeutic structure theory, and without that perspective, even if A-T split is adopted formally, it hardly functions effectively. Although the therapeutic structure theory developed in the practice of psychoanalytic therapy and psychoanalytic psychotherapy, it is also an important basic point of view in all other psychotherapeutic practices. It is a clinical activity that requires basic perspectives and procedures, such as constructive diagnostic interviews, the setting of a therapeutic structure based on those interviews, and adoption of A-T split in that structure. In this paper, A-T split was explained from the viewpoint of the therapeutic structure theory based on that fundamental principle. In addition, the course of treatment of a patient with relatively severe borderline personality disorder was introduced as a case report from the perspective of the administrator.

References

(1) Ekstein, Rudolf. 1952. "Structural Aspects of Psychotherapy". *Psychoanalytic Review*, Vol.39, No. 3: 222-229.

(2) Ikeda, Masakuni, Kinugasa, Takayuki, Taniyama, Junko. 2001. "High-function Developmental Disorder which are Discovered in Adulthood". Presented at the Semi-Annual Meeting of Department of Psychiatry and Neurosciences, Hiroshima University. (in Japanese)

(3) Iwasaki, Tetsuya, ed. 1990. *Therapeutic Structure Theory*. Tokyo: Iwasaki Academic Publisher. (in Japanese)

(4) Kinugasa, Takayuki. 1990. "Free Association and Frequency of Psychotherapy —From Experiences in Britain and Japan—". *The Japanese Journal of Psycho-analysis*, Vol. 33: 373-378. (in Japanese)

(5) Kinugasa, Takayuki. 1998. "What are Clinical Facts?". *Japanese Journal of Psycho-analysis*, Vol. 42: 17-22. (in Japanese), (Chapter 8 of this book (in English))

(6) Kinugasa, Takayuki. 2002. "Neutrality and Abstinence". *Japanese Journal of Psycho-analysis*, Vol. 46: 143-150. (in Japanese), (Chapter 9 of this book (in English))

(7) Kinugasa, Takayuki. 2004. "Borderline Personality Disorder and Developmental Disorder —About Layered-Clothes Syndrome—".

Japanese Journal of Psychiatric Treatment, Vol. 19: 693-699. (in Japanese)

(8) Okonogi, Keigo. 1990. "Introduction of the Therapeutic Structure Theory". In *Therapeutic Structure Theory*, edited by Tetsuya Iwasaki, 1-46. Tokyo: Iwasaki Academic Publisher. (in Japanese)

(9) Okonogi, Keigo. 1981. "Therapeutic Structure and Transference". *Japanese Journal of Psycho-analysis*, Vol. 26: 109-119. (in Japanese)

(10) Sekita, Kumi, Ikeda, Masakuni, Kinugasa, Takayuki., et al. 2005. "High-function Developmental Disorder in Postpubertal Patients with Diverse Psychic Symptoms —Layered-Clothes Syndrome—". *Japanese Journal of Psychoanalytical Psychiatry*, Vol. 1: 86-93. (in Japanese)

[2009. *Japanese Journal of Psychotherapy*, Vol. 35, No. 4.]

CHAPTER 14

THOSE THAT CONSTITUTE PSYCHOANALYSIS: FREE ASSOCIATION, NEUTRALITY AND FREE-FLOATING ATTENTION

1. Introduction

Here, I would like to explain the themes that form the basis of psychoanalysis. That is, I would like to talk about the basics of the therapeutic structure of psychoanalysis, the free association method, neutrality, and free-floating attention.

At the clinical site, which is the core of psychoanalysis, what Freud developed (e.g., the therapeutic setting, basic rules, basic pathology, basic theoretical perspectives, the therapist's attention points and viewpoints for understanding, and basic techniques for interpretation) are currently still the fundamentals of psychoanalysis. It can be said that psychoanalysis has now become more minute because treatment targets have gone through changes and theories including the developmental theory, anxiety theory, and structural theory have further developed and been performed. However, most of the frameworks of those basic ideas are composed of what Freud established during his lifetime. This is astonishing and indicates how revolutionary Freud's ideas were and how much they have provided important methods and perspectives for understanding the human mind.

At clinical sites in the Western countries and Japan, Freud's ideas are applied to once-or-twice-a-week psychoanalytic psychotherapy and other therapies. The Japan Psychoanalytical Association plays a primary role in conducting them in Japan. It can be understood that the therapies are based on a modified version of the therapeutic structure described below.

About 100 years ago, Freud stated in "Lines of Advance in Psychoanalytic Therapy" (24) that Freud himself had no choice but to treat only the wealthy due to social and historical circumstances, but the time would come in the future when psychoanalysis would be provided to the low-income masses under state compensation. He said that when the time comes, it might be a simplified version, but even if the therapeutic structure is changed, the core would be the knowledge and basic methods obtained from psychoanalysis. In fact, apart from the United States and South America, Western European countries, Oceania, and Canada adequately provide psychoanalytic psychotherapy with national insurance. In Japan, medical insurance guarantees are still insufficient and psychoanalytic psychotherapy that charge expensive costs is being conducted to a considerable extent. Is it that the time which Freud predicted is coming to Japan?

2. Therapeutic structure of psychoanalytic therapy—Discovery of the free association method

The answer for the question "What is psychoanalysis?" will be "It has a unique therapeutic structure. For the basic setting, the therapist will use a couch and the free association method and maintain discretion as a doctor based on a free-associative listening attitude (free-floating attention), neutrality and abstinence rules, and the ethical code." Furthermore, the goal of the treatment is to obtain much information from the patient, and clarify and raise awareness of the patient's unconscious pain and conflict in such a setting.

Although there are various concepts for them, the basic settings and viewpoints have been maintained until now, and it is an important task for clinicians to grasp the true clinical meaning of the basic techniques and viewpoints. For that purpose, it is crucial to know the beginning of such concepts and techniques and what kind of transition the historical meaning and significance have gone through. Understanding how they have been handed down to, understood and carried out by current therapists and how they have evolved and changed in daily clinical practice are also important tasks for a therapist.

The basic form of current psychoanalytic clinical practice was established in a relatively early state from around the eve to the dawn of psychoanalysis. The first phase was from the middle of 1880s to 1896, from the time when Freud was searching the pathology of and treatment for patients with hysteria through hypnosis, to the time when he developed the free association method from the patients' claim as a hint. The second phase was from 1897 to 1919, when Freud abandoned the trauma theory in 1897 and began advocating the drive theory. He discovered the method of dream interpretation and applied it to clinical practice and self-analysis, but it took more than 20 years to gradually clarify the structure of time and space. The third phase was from 1920 to the death of Freud in 1939. Basically, there was not much change in the therapeutic structure, and Freud advocated the theories including the instinct theory and the structure theory of id-ego-super-ego. Psychoanalysis after Freud's death entered the fourth phase, and flows of many schools such as the ego psychology school, Kleinian school, British independence group, self-psychology school, interpersonal relation school arose and have continued to the present. However, the basic settings, techniques, and the framework of the theoretical viewpoint and other features have been passed down up to the present.

Here, I would like to give an overview of the relationship between the central method of psychoanalysis and perspectives, focusing on Freud's cases and treatment structures, the history of the development of the free association method, and the current standing position.

(1) The era of research on hysteria: From hypnotic treatment to the discovery of the free association method [(10)]

a. Era of hypnosis era: Until the mid-1880s

Anna O. was a patient treated by J. Breuer. The therapeutic structure for her treatment has received little attention. Whenever requested, Breuer would make house visits and hypnotize the patient at the patient's home since he found that releasing the patient's emotions in various scenes in a hypnotic state was effective in eliminating symptoms (Catharsis therapy). Patient Anna began to request house visits many times a day, and Breuer visited each time and conducted treatment. Eventually, Anna O. began to develop symptoms such as intense transference love and a delusion of childbirth. This astonished Breuer and made him discontinue treatment and withdraw from studies on hysteria. In the case of Anna O, although there was a peculiar therapeutic structure, Breuer himself was only interested in the therapeutic effect of the catharsis method in hypnosis, and had no consideration on the significance of the therapeutic structure and transference relationship.

b. Freud: From the era of hypnosis to trial and error [(10)]

Even after Breuer withdrew from clinical research on hysteria, Freud continued to work alone to establish a treatment method. It is unknown how much attention Freud paid to matters such as time, place, and frequency then.

Freud was interested in, from his experiences including catharsis treatment, the idea that the core of hysteria's pathology was amnesia of the traumatic experience which was repressed in the topographical unconsciousness (concept of defence). He hypnotized patients for catharsis treatment with a central goal to eliminate the patient's symptoms by awakening the memory of the traumatic experience in the unconscious world. However, Freud discovered that symptoms recurred in hypnosis treatment and that not all patients responded to hypnosis, and abandoned hypnosis because he felt he was not good at hypnotizing. Nevertheless, Freud explained the pathology of hysteria with unconsciousness and repression, and thought that it was an important point of view that symptoms improved if the patient recalled the unconscious traumatic experiences and became conscious of them. He then began to aim to evoke repressed traumatic events while keeping the patient awake without conducting hypnosis. Freud used the questioning method, the commanding method, and the forehead method. The "Studies on Hysteria" describes the course of the case patient in detail based on the patient's data obtained by these methods. At that time, Freud used the couch he had used for hypnosis and instructed the patient to lie down. However, it is unclear to what extent Freud took into consideration about the setting such as treatment time, frequency, and treatment location. It seems that Freud took little account of them.

c. Discovery of the free association method

As described in "Studies on Hysteria," when Freud was trying to promote the patient (Emmy von N) to recall memories by means of questioning, commanding, and the forehead method, Emmy asked Freud to stop interrupting and just listen and let her talk freely. Freud did not overlook the words, felt its advantages, and got the inspiration for the free association method. Since then, he applied it to many patients and considered this method to be the most effective way to promote unconscious recalling for the patients. In the early days, however, Freud used free association to pursue the meaning of the symptoms.

Freud then used free association as a primary means to elucidate the meaning of dreams and finally succeeded in doing so ("Irma Dream" (9), (11)). After that, Freud adopted the free association method centrally in dream analysis for self-analysis ("The Interpretation of Dream" (11), "Dora case" (12)). He, at last, attained a true free association method for the whole mind ("Ratman case" (14)). Since then, Freud adopted this couch and non-focused free association method for the rest of his life. The post-Freud analysts have also adopted this method to date.

Freud only cited his own empirical reason to show why he thought this method was superior. He just gave a personal reason saying it was painful and he could not secure his own mental freedom when he was stared at by the patient all day long. However, this expresses Freud's excellent observant eye, clinical practical purpose-oriented aspect, and his ability to intuitively grasp the essence of human beings. In fact, Freud had conducted the basic methods and theoretical perspectives of current psychoanalysis at therapeutic sites by expanding his unique "participant observation", integrating it with logical thinking, for his practical experience with patients as humane physical existences and their phenomena. Freud found out many things through the treatment site using clinical observation as a pillar. That is, people avoided pain and sought for pleasure, suppressed excessive anxiety and pain, and eliminated them from their consciousness, and symptoms symbolically indicated the pathological state of the mind.

(2) Establishment of the therapeutic structure and the free association method

Freud clearly stated that he applied free association in the Ratman case (14), and it can be seen that the specific features including the use of a couch, lying-down method, regular sessions (1 hour), 6-times-a-week frequency, position of the therapist behind the patient, the neutrality of the therapist (which is described below), and the specific therapeutic stance such as "free-floating attention", were basically established then for the spatiotemporal structure. In his treatises on techniques such as "Recommendations to Physicians Practicing Psychoanalysis" (16) and "Further Recommendations on the Technique of Psychoanalysis" (18), Freud gave a clear and detailed explanation on matters such as the therapeutic structure and the mental stance of the therapist. In addition, he elucidated in "Introductory Lectures on Psychoanalysis" (22), which was published around the same time, that the therapeutic structure had been established by then.

In these treatises, Freud stated very humbly that the policies and precautions in conducting psychoanalysis described there were the methods Freud personally considered best, and were not absolute, and that they should be devised by each therapist. However, in reality, Freud did not change the therapeutic structure and free association method using a couch for the rest of his life. Many psychoanalysts have also conducted clinical treatment since Freud's death, but they have not changed this basic setting and method. They are still the main therapeutic structure and techniques.

Through the clinical experiences observed in this therapeutic structure and free association method using a couch, all psychoanalytic theories and techniques have evolved. In other words, the importance of transference and acting-out, the importance of counter-transference and their therapeutic significances have developed. In addition, basic viewpoints, e.g., topographical theory (unconscious theory), drive theory, economic theory, developmental theory, anxiety/conflict theory, structural theory (id-ego-super-ego), object relation theory and adaptation theory, which are Freud's basic theories, have developed as a magnificent flow. They have been modified and developed with the times and the transition of treatment targets, but their importance as basic viewpoints have never faded.

Many psychoanalysts have continued to appreciate and adhere to the outstanding points of this therapeutic structure and free association technique. In that process, it has been indicated that what Freud created through his intuitive insight and persevering trial and error is an excellent method to observe human beings and is the most elaborate method to reveal unconscious activities.

3. Characteristics of Freud's basic thinking method

As for the explanation of why the human mind is made like this and why his method was the optimal treatment method, Freud just cited the effectiveness in his trial-and-error clinical experiences. It seems that he did not try to face the theoretical questions himself. He intended to just maintain the what-he-called scientific method and describe the characteristics of what he observed in his concrete involvement with his patients as somatic beings. It seems that he always kept in mind the induction method of creating a concept that explains the characteristics observed at clinical sites, e.g., "Pathologies such as hysteria are pathologies of forgotten memories," and "There exists an unconsciousness in the mind."

Not only in his profound metapsychology presented in his papers including "Project for a Scientific Psychology" (9), "The Interpretation of Dreams, Chapter VII" (11), "Instincts and Their Vicissitudes" (20), but also in his instinct anxiety theory and explanation of the mind's unconscious world, Freud thoroughly focused on how observed facts should be explained from cytological and biological perspectives, and from what point of view they should be seen. He gave little direction to consider the philosophical principles of human existence.

Freud did not try much to approach the explanatory world of the philosophical principle theory or ontology which asks "why" about the phenomenon. In fact, he declared himself that he consciously avoided the world of philosophy. It seems that he chose not to enter the world of doubts on the existence principle of the state of mind.

Bion et al. appear to have tried to work their way into the world of ontology (2), (3), (4), (6), but basically, Bion also attempted to clarify the mental situation based on clinical experiences and observation including thinking disorder in treatment of psychosis, indistinguishability between reality and hallucinations in psychotic transferences and unidentifiability between reality and psychic reality (5). Nevertheless, Bion stepped into the world of ontology far more than Freud, and as a result, developed a world common to the philosophical thinking of ontology, which can be said to be an extremely esoteric semiotic ontology. This was what Freud was trying to keep away as far he could.

It seems that Freud had foreseen that understanding and explaining the world of the apriori existence principle would be an extremely difficult task. He tried not to enter the principle field; e.g., what the mind is, why emotions exist, and why humans have a mind. For example, in physics, it is still extremely difficult to answer the fundamental questions of what the universe is, what gravity and weight are, and what light is. Actual academic progress is based on observation. There is daily progress and new discoveries in the directions and fields which try to clarify what kind of characteristics there are in the cosmic activity, gravity and light through observation and purpose-oriented logics. Psychoanalysis has a similar direction, and Freud called it a scientific method and stated that it was not oriented to philosophy.

4. Characteristic and advantages of the free association method using a couch

The expression form using the free association method with a couch, which was intuitively selected by Freud, has been supported empirically to be the most appropriate method for patients' self-expression up until now, basically without being changed. This is probably because there is something suitable in the method for expressing the human mind, especially the unconscious world. In the history of psychoanalysis, questions such as "Why are the facts and methods which Freud empirically and intuitively observed and devised in clinical practice the most appropriate? ", and "What properties and characteristics do they connote?" have often arose. These questions have developed as an inductive explanatory concept based on experience. The free association method using a couch is one of the typical examples.

It has been empirically considered that free association performed while the patient is lying on a couch is most suitable for the patient to express his/her unconsciousness and the therapist to observe him/her, however, the reason has not been clearly answered. Nevertheless, the advantages and characteristics of its therapeutic structure have often been discussed. They can be summarized as the following opinions [(29), (32), (35), (46), (47), (50), (53)].

(1) The relationship between the patient and the therapist is unequal. The patient seeks help and is, in a sense, subordinate to the therapist. This is a fundamental and important factor in the free association method.

Furthermore, in a situation where a spatiotemporal structure is frequently provided and a homeostasis is guaranteed, the basic structure is that the patient lies on a couch and the therapist listens in a sitting position behind the patient's head. The free association method is guaranteed and protected in that environment. However, when the patient gives free association, it is considered that the patient has a paradoxical experience that he/she does not experience on a daily basis.

a In situations where time and space are set and the patient is instructed to lie down on a couch, the patient is left in a defenceless and helpless state, is forcedly deprived of freedom by an authority, looked down from above, and is in a restrained state. This is similar to the relationship between parents and children that incites castration anxiety and envy. Being instructed to give free association in such a state is compulsory, however, the patient is guaranteed his/her freedom of expression only in that state.

b Another possibility is that this constant therapeutic relationship is like a situation of a mother-child relationship. The patient's recumbent state on a couch is similar to a state of an infant, whose motor function is still weak, lying in a cradle. This state and the relationship themselves may stimulate the patient's infantile mentality and lead the patient to their unconscious world. Being forced to give free associations in that situation means that the patient is asked for free self-expression and also is receiving strict discipline. However, it also creates a condition similar to the infantile experience under the mother's care and protection. In that sense, it is a structure suitable for the patient and the therapist to pay attention to the infantile aspect of the patient's self.

Okonogi explained the situation when the patient's disposition toward such therapeutic structure was manifested with the concept of "structural transference" [(48)].

(2) About the paradox of free-association itself: The free association method has an essential paradox, that is, the patient is instructed to speak freely in an atmosphere where the therapist is receptive and neutral and takes an attentive attitude to listen. Free association is free within that condition; however, treatment is not guaranteed unless that instruction is followed. Furthermore, it is by no means free or easy to speak in free association. In other words, the patient follows the "pleasure-principle" of being able to express freely, but on the other hand, encounters abstinence, the "discomfort principle" and the "reality principle". The patient is encouraged to speak in a primitive and regressive world, where the patient's freedom is limited to only language, and their physical activity is also restricted.

(3) For the patients to give free association, they must split themself. On the one hand, their infantile world is stimulated and they can regress

freely and fulfil their world of narcissism, but they also have to tell their painful world and experience strong emotions and resistance. It is also a world of infantile satisfaction where the patients win recognition from the therapist by cooperating with the therapist to carry them out. On the other hand, as such a regressive state deepens, the patients' secondary function increases. Patients work with the therapist to improve their self-observing ability and enhance their linguistic expressive ability. These become possible in a specific protective environment based on the therapist's neutrality.

(4) This structure and free association method are something that highlights the origin of human relationships and communication. This probably is currently the optimal therapeutic structure for the therapist and the patient to look together at the interaction between the unconscious world of the patient and the unconscious world of the therapist, which is what Freud aimed.

(5) Bion described the therapist-patient relationship in this structuring with the model of the mother-child relationship and explained it with the concept of container/contained [(2), (3), (6)]. The baby expresses its experience freely with emotion, and excludes and throws the unbearable anxiety experience into the mother. The mother introjects it, grasps its meaning by reverie, that is, the α function, and returns it in a form that the baby can accept. The baby introjects this and accumulates its experiences in its mind as meaningful things. In this myriad of repetitions, the baby creates a meaningful world of self in its mind.

Bion believed that this container/contained mother-infant relationship was developed in patient-therapist communication within the therapeutic structure and therapeutic relationship of psychoanalysis. The therapist would make full use of his/her reverie, that is, the α function, to read the meaning of anxiety, transference, and defence and other movements of the mind expressed in the content of the patient's free association, and give interpretations to the patient. He considered that repetition and accumulation of this process would promote the development and integration of the patient's mind.

Based on this perspective, Bion theoretically developed his idea to a general communication theory. He highlighted the essence of human communication and created a stir in the essential question of how people can perceive and understand other people's mind. He then discussed the relativity of communication and said that the absolute truth in the unconsciousness of the mind cannot be directly touched neither by ourselves nor by others. Bion discussed the relativity of human communication, that is, the absolute truth is always conveyed as indirect symbolic expressions, and even the speaker him/herself cannot directly know his/her own absolute truth, and the recipient, another person, has no choice but to infer the truth from the symbolically communicated content.

5. Subsequent transitions in therapeutic targets and the free association method

Free association using a couch has subsequently played a central role as a therapeutic structure, however, its role has been questioned with the transition of times, especially when new therapeutic targets appeared.

(1) Treatment of psychosis: Discord with K. Abraham [(1)]

As Freud made clear in Schreber's case study [(15)], patients with psychoses such as schizophrenia and manic-depressive illness withdraw libido from their object and are in an objectless narcissistic world. Therefore, Freud thought that those patients could not cause transferences and would not be subject to psychoanalysis. He thus argued that a couch was not to be used, the free association method was not applicable and also interpretations should not be made. Freud thought that if psychotherapy was to be conducted, the technique should be modified and changed to supportive care. Freud's disciple, Federn [(7)], conducted a psychotherapeutic study on schizophrenia. Federn followed Freud's idea and tried to help patients with a modified psychotherapy focusing on maternal supportive care. A guideline which applies this modified technique was passed on mainly to North American psychoanalysts [(28), (51), (55)].

K. Abraham boldly worked on psychoanalytic treatment in patients with manic-depressive illness and considered their pathological fixation point was in the pathological condition of 6-month-old babies' disposition (in the 1910s). He adopted the free association method using a couch and conducted therapy centred on interpreting transferences. He further subdivided the oral stage, the anal stage, and phallic stage of Freud's development theory, and considered that the pathological fixation point of manic-depressive disease was the conflict between drive and object relations from the late oral stage to the early anal stage. While he was working on his clinical studies, he experienced intense discord with Freud. However, Freud came to be greatly influenced by Abraham when discussing pathology in the study of manic-depressive illness [(23)]. It became the basis for Freud's remarkable leaps to narcissism, object incorporation, object loss theory, super-ego theory and other theories in the 1910s and 1920s.

As mentioned above, Abraham advocated the idea that disorders of the early object relations in 0-year-olds was the fixation point for manic-depressive illness and paranoia, and greatly influenced Klein. It can be said that Abraham is one of the first proponents of contemporary object relations theory.

(2) A new assessment of the free association method by Melanie Klein

Since I, the author, am an analyst influenced by the Kleinian school, I would like to explain the new therapeutic targets in that trend and how the free association method developed.

a Psychoanalysis for extremely young children

It can be said that the advent of Melanie Klein brought a new perspective and infused new breath into the free association method. At this time too, the encounter with new treatment targets led to innovative perspectives and theoretical progress. The free association method was at the centre of this change, and made significant advance [(36), (37), (38), (39), (40), (41)].

From the 1920s, Klein began working on psychoanalysis in children with Anna Freud. In "The Case of Little Hans" [(13)], Sigmund Freud proposed a guiding principle that the target for children's psychoanalysis should be children who had formed an inner world after the Oedipus complex, which comes around at the age around 3 to 5, and whose language function was competent enough for the use of the free association method. Furthermore, according to Freud, since the inner world is not formed yet in children below the age of 3, they have no ability to generate transferences and their language function is still immature. Thus, he thought treatment for little children should be focused on guidance for their parents. For the following 10 years, psychoanalysis for children had rarely been the subject of research. Anna Freud followed her father's policy and began psychoanalysis focusing on verbal free association in children over the age of 5.

Klein, on the other hand, accumulated experience in treating slightly older children under S. Ferenczi in the late 1910s. However, she began to work on clinical research of psychoanalysis for very young children below the age of 3 under Abraham in Berlin in 1921. This was when her teacher, Abraham, was conducting psychoanalytic study on manic-depressive illness and evolving his theory on pathology and development of 6-month-old disposition in young children.

He recommended Klein to study psychoanalytical therapy for very young children below the age of 3, and it seems that he had felt the need to confirm the importance of the 6-month-old disposition in infants. Following that recommendation, Klein began treating very young children aged 2 to 3 years. There, she faced young children with psychotic symptoms, autistic tendencies, severe night terrors, intense compulsive behaviours, and conduct disorders, who could barely talk. Klein prepared a number of toys, painting tools, and other stuff, and observed their play. She discovered that their play presented many symbolic meanings. She then applied the technique of dream interpretation and realized that the children's play symbolically represented their unconscious world. She then came to think that "children's play has expressive power comparable to adults' free association method using language". Since then, through play therapy (free association) for the children she treated, Klein came to understand the unconscious world of 0-year-old children. This greatly overturned Freud's previous idea that an inner world was not yet formed in children younger than 3 years old, and evoked much debate. However, it was a magnificent breakthrough which led to the dawn of current psychoanalysis.

Klein revealed the pathological conditions of 0-year-old children. The essential features are: i) The unconscious world of 2 to 3 year old children is composed of the 0-year-old dispositions; ii) It is a world in which internal part-objects and whole objects are intricately active; iii) Central emotions and anxieties are persecutory anxiety and depressive anxiety, and it is a world where aggression and sadism are predominant; iv) Primitive defence mechanisms are seen where splitting, projection, incorporation, denial, and omnipotence are active; v) These inner worlds of 0-year-olds are transferred to the therapist in analytical treatment, and the therapist can provide therapeutic assistance by verbally interpreting the transferences.

Klein did not use a couch for children's play therapy and regarded the entire consultation room as a place of expression. She regarded the entire activity of children, including play with toys, drawing, and actions, as something that freely expressed the children's inner world, equivalent to adult's free associations using language.

This was something that overturned the then-established theory of psychoanalysis. Although Freud himself did not approve it, Abraham and E. Jones from London, where Klein later emigrated, strongly supported it. This new application and deployment of the free association method made a revolution in the world of psychoanalysis. It was initially confined to Berlin and London, but eventually came to influence throughout North America in the 1980s. Currently, the activity of the inner world of 0-year-olds and the pathological importance are recognized by psychoanalysts all over the world.

b Psychoanalytic study on adult manic-depressive illness and schizophrenia by Klein

From the 1930s, Klein decided to take over Abraham's research and began practicing psychoanalytic treatment for adult manic-depressive illness. At that time, Klein confirmed that the pathology of the 6-month-old infant disposition, which Abraham advocated, was at the centre of the inner conflict in manic-depressive patients, and proposed the concept of the "depressive position" [(41), (42)]. Klein's revolutionary ideas and techniques were manifested when she reversed a maxim and declared then that "Adult free association using language is comparable to children's play." In short, Klein innovatively renovated the perspective on the understanding of adult free association from the traditional one. Briefly, what is expressed in adult free association is influenced by unconscious phantasies that are currently active, similar to children's play. The unconscious phantasy activities, motives and other matters are indirectly and symbolically expressed in the selection and composition of the materials and stories. It is an application of dream interpretation, in which free association at the time of awakening is regarded as manifest dreams, and the current state of the unconscious phantasies is regarded as latent dreams. Klein considered that free associations of the conscious world were expressions of unconscious phantasies that were distortedly expressed by mechanisms such as symbolization, displacement, and condensation.

The role of the therapist is to listen attentively to the free associations and read the unconscious activities in the expressions. It is to read and interpret the relationship between the unconscious themes and transferences (especially the unconscious transference relationships). On that account, therapists read the unconscious world by making full use of even the therapist's normal counter-transferences.

From the 1940s, Klein conducted psychoanalytic studies on schizophrenia with Kleinian scholars such as H. Rosenfeld [(49)], H. Segal [(50)], and Bion [(5)]. She used the free association method with a couch at this time too, and revealed that patients with schizophrenia have a pathology of a 3-month-old baby's disposition. She then proposed the concept of the paranoid-schizoid position [(42)].

As described above, the free association method is a core clinical method in psychoanalysis. The method has become what it is today after the evolution of its meaning and the transition of its treatment targets and therapeutic techniques.

6. Basic stance of therapists: Neutrality, free-floating attention

Next, I would like to describe the therapeutic structural stance of the therapist.

In response to structurally instructing the patient to give free associations on a couch, the therapist also faces the patient in a unique stance. Structurally, the therapist sits in a chair by the patient's head on the couch and listens to the patient's free associations. At that time, the therapist is also expected to maintain various conventions. The true purposes are to promote the patient's free association, to keep the therapist's state of mind constant, and to correctly read and respond to the unconscious meanings.

(1) Neutrality and abstinence [(33), (16)]

Freud advocated neutrality as the basic attitude of the therapist. This means that the therapist takes a neutral attitude, stance, and perspective. Externally, the therapist should be modest, flatten his/her mind and behave like a screen that reflects the patient's emotions and thoughts. The voice intonation and facial expressions (although the patient always cannot see them) should not be affected by the therapist's counter-transference.

In addition, the therapist should maintain an attitude of acceptance and attentive listening, with discretion as a humble therapist, while refraining from moral judgment and personal commentary on the content of the patient's free association. These attitudes promote free association of the patient and enhance the listening ability of the therapist.

Furthermore, there are strict prohibitions. As abstinence rules, it is prohibited to satisfy the patient's drives, and the therapist must refrain from satisfying his/her own drives and desires. Socially, as ethical codes, the confidentiality of the patient's personal information must be kept, and the therapist must not make bad use of the patient personally, must not sexually harass or physically abuse the patient and must not personally use the patient's information.

There are very practical reasons and policies aimed to promote the patient's free associations and properly perceive and understand their unconscious manifestations in the background of maintaining this neutrality, these abstinence rules, and these ethical codes as an expert. Freud's basic therapeutic goal, that is to make conscious the unconsciousness, was maintained throughout his life from the beginning of his research on hysteria.

Freud believed that counter-transference was not desirable and would be a hindrance to treatment because it distorted and prevented the understanding of the patient's free association. He also thought it was important for the therapist to clear away his/her counter-transference caused by unresolved conflicts as much as possible through training analysis and self-analysis. By the way, around 1950, P. Heiman proposed the concept of normal counter-transference, and since then it has developed as an important technical concept.

(2) "Free-floating attention" [16], [18], [54], [45]

Freud argued that the therapist should remain neutral, have a state of mind like a screen that reflects the patient's mind, and deal with the patient's problems as dispassionately as a surgeon. On the other hand, he stated that it was essential to maintain a state, using neutrality, where the therapist could sensitively catch the communication from the patient's unconsciousness, just like a telephone receiver.

In this way, the goal for therapists is to sensitively catch what is transmitted from the patient's unconsciousness by adopting the free association method to make it easier for the patient's unconscious activities to be exposed and maintaining neutrality and free unbiased sensitivity.

Freud became aware of the importance of "free-floating attention" when he realized the importance of unfocused true free association by a patient. By the time of the "Ratman case" in 1907, it seems that he had already adopted the method, and by the time he presented some of his techniques from 1912 to 1914, he clearly considered it to be an important attitude of the therapist. This is, so to speak, internal neutrality. The "free-floating attention" keeps the therapist in a state where he/she is not affected by elements such as his/her personal interests, attention points, and memories, and creates a state where his/her thoughts and fantasies can be freely active. He thought it would enable the therapist's unconscious receiver to perceive the patient's unconscious communication more sensitively.

Furthermore, around the same time, the importance of understanding counter-transference was emphasized, and individual analysis and training analysis came to be required to ameliorate the therapist's individual unresolved neurotic conflicts and blind spots as much as possible.

This "free-floating attention" is still considered as the therapist's basic mental stance. This is an extremely clinically practical concept, but for the therapist to master it and acquire it as a clinically humane concept for execution, the therapist is required to accumulate many clinical experiences, receive much guidance from experts, and continue polishing his/her skills with colleagues. Later, Bion [6] reconsidered Freud's specific mental stance of the therapist, and expressed it with a phrase "no memory, no desire".

(3) The free association method and free-floating attention

The strict and characteristic structuring of dialogue and interaction between the patient and the therapist is the most elaborate and sophisticated method to aim for a total mind-to-mind communication, from the unconscious world to the conscious world.

Psychoanalytic theories and techniques are based on overall communication ranging from unconsciousness to overall conscious communication between the patient and the therapist in this setting. Therapists have worked on the patients, given considerations on the obtained information in a practice-oriented concrete situation and aimed for further techniques and theoretical development with a central goal to correspond to the observation items and unconsciousness based on participant observation.

Once again, Freud's important clinical technical perspectives were mostly born from his clinical trials and errors, and have been chosen as the most therapeutically viable methods by his delicate and keen intuition. In the background, there was a clear point of view that aiming to become conscious of the patient's unconsciousness was the most important therapeutic goal. As for the theoretical discussion, while empirically mastering the therapeutic importance and effectiveness of those phenomena, Freud also gave an enormous amount of clinical or metapsychological considerations thinking why they are so and what kind of clinical significance they have. This Freud's hands-on approach is quite specific to psychoanalysis. When he was asked what psychoanalysis was, he replied that it was something that delt with resistance and transferences. This answer is premised on the background therapeutic structure and represents his true value as a practitioner.

(4) Problem of neutrality [33]

Historically, the school that focused on the therapist's behaviour and screen-like attitude where the therapist does not show emotions among the clinical significance of neutrality was the ego psychology school (classical psychoanalysis). In practice, the analysts in that position seemed to aim for complete passiveness and emotional blockade, and were said to be very careful in their interpretations. As K. Menninger suggests in his book on techniques, patients are exposed to frustration against the attitude of the therapist who hardly shows reaction at the therapeutic site based on the free association method using a couch and regression is promoted. It is considered that early infantile associations are recalled more in that situation.

It is said that it was M. Kohut who criticized and disagreed with this issue of neutrality, arguing that the therapist's empathic attitude and words and behaviour were therapeutically important. He established self-psychology, which is still developing as a theory of intersubjectivity.

On the other hand, in the UK's object relation theory (in a broad sense), although it was considered as a modest attitude, the issue of the neutral attitude did not head towards extreme emotional blockage. It is much related to the difference in technical approaches to the content of the free association method. As mentioned above, the unconsciousness of the moment is expressed by phenomena such as symbolization, displacement, and condensation in adult's free association, just like child's play, and Klein insisted that the therapist should grasp the activity of the unconscious phantasies and proactively perform transference interpretations. Therefore, the therapist thinks and intervenes proactively maintaining sensitivity to the unconsciousness under the concept of neutrality and free-floating attention. During the treatment sessions, the therapist will have many opportunities to express his/her emotions and human attitude through active interpretations of what he/she understands and, in a sense, by how he/she intervenes. As for the issue of neutrality, what came to be emphasized is that the therapist has to be modest and adopt a neutral attitude towards his/her sensibilities and thoughts in order to refine and maintain his/her sensitivities. Thus, the issue of the so-called "non-responding therapists as if they had expressionless Noh masks on", which has been discussed in American ego psychology, did not become a problematic issue in the UK.

7. Conclusion

Here, under the title of "Those that Constitute Psychoanalysis," I tried clarifying the significance of psychoanalysis as the most basic place for interaction in regards to the free association method for patients, and the neutrality and free-floating attention of the therapist.

The indefinite conversation that unfolds between the patient, who gives information through communication using the free association method under a specific structure and conditions described above, and the therapist, who has prepared a neutral attitude and sensitivity to receive the information (free-floating attention), is the fundamental basis of psychoanalysis. The process how the therapist judges and thinks about it, grasps the activity of unconsciousness, and holds a certain degree of conviction about the patient's current condition is iterated at the site of psychoanalytic therapy.

The question of how the patient-therapeutic relationship changes at the therapeutic site is still a major task to be answered. In actual treatment practice, there are still many difficult questions that need to be asked: What kind of basic viewpoint does the therapist have? What is the viewpoint like? Is it a conscious viewpoint or an unconscious viewpoint? and so on.

References

(1) Abraham, Karl. 1927. *Selected Papers of Karl Abraham, M.D.* London: Hogarth Press and the Institute of Psycho-analysis.

(2) Bion, Wilfred. 1962. *Learning from Experience*. London: Heinemann.

(3) Bion, Wilfred. 1963. *Elements of Psychoanalysis*. London: Heinemann.

(4) Bion, Wilfred. 1965. *Transformation*s. London: Heinemann.

(5) Bion, Wilfred. 1967. *Second Thoughts*. London: Heinemann.

(6) Bion, Wilfred. 1970/1977. "Attention and Interpretation". In *Seven Servants*. New York: Jason Aronson.

(7) Federn, Paul. 1953. *Ego Psychology and the Psychoses*. New York: Basic Books.

(8) Ferenczi, Sandor. 1994. *First Contributions to Psycho-Analysis*. London: Karnac Books.

(9) Freud, Sigmund. 1895. "Project for a Scientific Psychology". In *Standard Edition*, Vol. 1. London: Hogarth Press.

(10) Freud, Sigmund. 1985. "Studies on Hysteria". In *Standard Edition*, Vol. 2. London: Hogarth Press.

(11) Freud, Sigmund. 1900. "The Interpretation of Dreams". In *Standard Edition*, Vol.4-5. London: Hogarth Press.

(12) Freud, Sigmund. 1905. "Fragment of an Analysis of a Case of Hysteria". In *Standard Edition*, Vol. 7. London: Hogarth Press.

(13) Freud, Sigmund. 1909. "Analysis of a Phobia in a Five-Year-Old Boy". In *Standard Edition*, Vol. 10. London: Hogarth Press.

(14) Freud, Sigmund. 1909. "Notes upon a Case of Obsessional Neurosis". In *Standard Edition*, Vol. 10. London: Hogarth Press.

(15) Freud, Sigmund. 1911. "Psycho-analytic Notes on an Autobiographical Account of a Case of Paranoia (Dementia Paranoides)". In *Standard Edition*, Vol. 12: 3-82. London: Hogarth Press.

(16) Freud, Sigmund. 1912. "Recommendation to Physicians Practicing Psychoanalysis". In *Standard Edition*, Vol. 12. London: Hogarth Press.

(17) Freud, Sigmund. 1912. "The Dynamics of Transference". In *Standard Edition*, Vol. 12. London: Hogarth Press.

(18) Freud, Sigmund. 1913. "Further Recommendations on the Technique of Psychoanalysis, I: On Beginning the Treatment". In *Standard Edition*, Vol. 12. London: Hogarth Press.

(19) Freud, Sigmund. 1914. "On the History of Psychoanalytic Movement". In *Standard Edition*, Vol. 14. London: Hogarth Press.

(20) Freud, Sigmund. 1915. "Instincts and Their Vicissitudes". In *Standard Edition*, Vol. 14. London: Hogarth Press.
(21) Freud, Sigmund. 1917. "Further Recommendations on the Technique of Psychoanalysis, II: Remembering, Repeating and Working-Through". In *Standard Edition*, Vol. 12. London: Hogarth Press.
(22) Freud, Sigmund. 1916-1917. "Introductory Lectures on Psycho-Analysis". In *Standard Edition*, Vol. 15-16. London: Hogarth Press.
(23) Freud, Sigmund. 1917. "Mourning and Melancholia". In *Standard Edition*, Vol. 14. London: Hogarth Press.
(24) Freud, Sigmund. 1919. "Lines of Advance in Psychoanalytic Therapy". In *Standard Edition*, Vol. 17. London: Hogarth Press.
(25) Freud, Sigmund. 1920. "A Note on the Prehistory of the Technique of Analysis". In *Standard Edition*, Vol. 18. London: Hogarth Press.
(26) Freud, Sigmund. 1925. "An Autobiographical Study". In *Standard Edition*, Vol. 20. London: Hogarth Press.
(27) Freud, Sigmund. 1940. "An Outline of Psychoanalysis". In *Standard Edition*, Vol. 23. London: Hogarth Press.
(28) Fromm-Reichmann, Frieda. 1959. *Psychoanalysis and Psychotherapy. Selected Papers of Frieda Fromm-Reichmann*. Chicago: The University of Chicago Press.
(29) Green, Andrè. 2000. "The Central Phobic Position: A New Formulation of The Free Association Method". *International Journal of Psycho-Analysis*, Vol. 81: 429-451.
(30) Heimann, Paula. 1950. "On Counter-Transference". *International Journal of Psycho-Analysis*, Vol. 31: 81-84.
(31) Hoffer, Axel, and Youngren, Virginia R. 2004. "Is Free Association still at the core of Psychoanalysis?". *International Journal of Psycho-Analysis*, Vol. 85: 1489-1492.
(32) Hoffman, Irwin. Z. 2006. "The Myths of Free Association and the Potentials of the Analytic Relationship". *International Journal of Psycho-Analysis*, Vol. 87: 43-61.
(33) Kanzer, Mark. 1972. "Superego Aspects of Free Association and the Fundamental Rule". *Journal of the American Psychoanalytic Association*, Vol. 20: 246-266.
(34) Kinugasa, Takayuki. 1995. "Current Movement of Modern Kleinians". In *Present of Psychoanalysis,* Extra Issue, L'esprit d'aujourd'hui. Tokyo: Shibundo Publishing (in Japanese)
(35) Kinugasa, Takayuki. 2002. "Neutrality and Discipline of Abstinence". *The Japanese Journal of Psycho-Analysis,* Vol. 46, No. 2: 143-150 (in Japanese) (Chapter 9 of this book (in English))

(36) Klein, Melanie. 1926. "The Psychological Principles of Early Analysis". *International Journal of Psycho-Analysis,* Vol. 8: 25-37.
(37) Klein, Melanie. 1927. "Symposium on child analysis". *International Journal of Psycho-Analysis,* Vol. 8: 339-370.
(38) Klein, Melanie. 1928. "Early stages of the Oedipus conflict". *International Journal of Psycho-Analysis,* Vol. 9: 167-180.
(39) Klein, Melanie 1929. "Personification in the Play of Children". *International Journal of Psycho-Analysis,* Vol. 10: 193-204.
(40) Klein, Melanie. 1932/1975. "Psychoanalysis of Children". In *The Writings of Melanie Klien*, Vol. 2. London: Hogarth Press.
(41) Klein, Melanie. 1935. "A Contribution to the Psychogenesis of Manic-Depressive States". *International Journal of Psycho-Analysis,* Vol. 16: 145-174.
(42) Klein, Melanie. 1940/1975. "Mourning and Its Relation to Manic-Depressive States". In *The Writings of Melanie Klien,* Vol. 1: 344-369. London: Hogarth Press.
(43) Klein, Melanie. 1946/1952. "Notes on Some Schizoid Mechanisms". In *Developments in Psychoanalysis*: 292-320. London: Hogarth Press.
(44) Kris, Anton O. 1983. "The Analyst's Conceptual Freedom in the Method of Free Association". *International Journal of Psycho-Analysis,* Vol. 64: 407-411.
(45) Langen, Robert. 1997. "On Free-Floating Attention". *Psychoanalytic Dialogues*, Vol. 7: 819-839.
(46) Loewenstein, Rudolph M. 1963. "Some Consideration on Free Association". *Journal of the American Psychoanalytic Association*, Vol. 11: 451-473.
(47) McDermott, Virginia A. 2003. "Is Free Association Still Fundamental?". *Journal of the American Psychoanalytic Association*, Vol. 51: 1349-1356.
(48) Okonogi, Keigo. 1990. "Introduction to the Theory of Therapeutic Structure". In *Theory of Therapeutic Structure*, edited by Tetsuya Iwasaki, 1-46. Tokyo: Iwasaki Academic Publisher. (in Japanese)
(49) Rosenfeld, Herbert. 1947/1965. "Analysis of a Schizophrenic State with Depersonalization". In *Psychotic States*, 13-33. London: Hogarth Press.
(50) Rosner, Stanley. 1973. "On the Nature of Free Association". *Journal of the American Psychoanalytic Association*, Vol. 21: 558-575.
(51) Searles, Harold F. 1963: *Collected Papers on Schizophrenia and related subjects*. London: Hogarth Press.
(52) Segal, Hanna. 1981. *The Work of Hanna Segal: A Kleinian Approach*

to Clinical Practice. New York: Jason Aronson.
(53) Seidenberg, Henry. 1971. "The Basic Rule: Free Association—A Reconsideration". *Journal of the American Psychoanalytic Association*, Vol. 19: 98-109.
(54) Spence, Donald P. 1984. "Perils and Pitfalls of Free Floating Attention". *Contemporary Psychoanalysis*, Vol.20: 37-59.
(55) Sullivan, Harry. 1974. *Schizophrenia as a Human Process*. New York: Norton & Company.
(56) Teller, Virginia, and Dahl, Hartvig. 1986. "The Microstructure of Free Association". *Journal of the American Psychoanalytic Association*, Vol. 34: 763-798.
(57) Trosman, Harry. 1969. "The Cryptomnesic Fragment in the Discovery of Free Association". *Journal of the American Psychoanalytic Association*, Vol. 17: 489-510.

[2015. *The Japanese Journal of Psycho-Analysis*, Vol. 59, No. 1.]

CHAPTER 15

EVERYDAY ANALYSIS AND DREAM INTERPRETATION

1. Introduction

Everyday analysis is very closely associated with the clinical practice of dream interpretation. It is generally known that the number of dreams reported increases with the increase in the frequency of treatment, even in patients with the same level of pathology. Additionally, in everyday analysis, there are some patients who are in a state where they rarely talk about dreams and they can only provide extremely ordinary and concrete reports. It is pointed out that in such cases, severe pathology often exists. Such patients are patients with an extremely strong suppression and they hardly exhibit abilities of phantasy or imagination. They have a psychotic tendency; however, even if they are not psychotic, their symbolic function has not developed adequately. In many cases, they can only develop a world of concrete enactment with individuals they encounter in everyday life. Some of them also exhibit the 'layered-clothes syndrome'. Additionally, according to W. Bion, when the psychotic part of the personality is active, the patient has no ability to have dreams. Further, even when the patient reports something as a dream, it is often a psychotic experience that the patient has had during sleep.

Here, I would like to emphasize the importance of dream analysis in everyday analysis, and to introduce how the actuals and theories of dream analysis have developed from Freud to Kleinians, and to the theory of object relations. I will then report a case and highlight the importance of dream analysis in everyday analysis. Although I do not aim to compare and investigate the frequency of psychoanalytical psychotherapy and dream reports, the treatment frequency per week and the dream frequency, as well as the importance of the therapeutic significance, have a relatively proportional relationship.

First, I would like to briefly introduce S. Freud's dream theory, followed by the clinical practice and theories of dreams in contemporary Kleinians, and in the theory of object relations. Next, I will introduce actual dream reports and their interpretations in sessions of everyday analysis. I will present that the development of transferences and the dreams themselves act as a resistance, and emphasize the importance of dreams in everyday analysis.

2. Fundamental viewpoints of Freud's dream interpretation

Freud began working on the treatment of hysteria in the 1980's. At first he tried methods such as hypnosis, the ordering-to-remember method, and the pressure-to-forehead method. He later abandoned these methods because they were unsuccessful. Finally, he developed the free association method using a couch. The idea occurred to Freud when a patient told him that she wanted to speak freely while he was conducting various techniques such as suggesting and questioning. Freud conducted such sessions six times a week and kept doing so for the rest of his career considering this as the basic therapeutic structure for psychoanalysis. Everyday analysis became, and continues to be, the central methodology in psychoanalysis.

In such structure, Freud focused on the fact that many of the patients with neurosis reported dreams when he was treating them. Thus, he started putting efforts on developing a method to understand the meaning of dreams. He then succeeded in self-interpreting a dream that he had on July 23-24, 1895. It was a dream on his patient Irma; therefore, it is famous as 'Irma's dream'. His unique method of dream interpretation involved conducting free association for each element of the dream and understanding the true, unconscious meaning of the dream from the overall information of those associations. Freud then proposed the thesis "A dream is a fulfilment of a wish".

Subsequently, Freud interpreted many of his own dreams and his patients' dreams, and this method utilizing free association of dream elements became the fundamental process of dream analysis in psychoanalysis. He established the following fundamental concepts of dream theory, which he hardly modified thereafter: i) manifest dreams and latent dreams, and dream work; ii) censorship of dreams and condensation, displacement, symbolism; iii) fulfilment of a wish; iv) security of sleep, and meaning of anxiety dreams and nightmares v) primary process and secondary process; vi) secondary revision; vii) regression; and viii) dream from below and dream from above. Since these viewpoints are well known, their explanations will be omitted in this paper.

Freud presupposed the following viewpoints here: i) dreams have meanings, ii) a part of the mind is active and can possess wishes even during sleep, iii) wishes can be expressed in an iconic primitive form, iv) there is a part of mind which monitors these wishes, v) there is an action of mind which censors the dream and makes compromises using a complex mechanism such as displacement, condensation, and symbolism. These premises were refined by later Kleinians and object-relation theorists.

3. Characteristics of M. Klein's dream interpretation

(1) M. Klein reported many dreams. Most of her case reports focused on dream analysis. Klein and the researchers introduced later in this paper used everyday analysis as the basis for their studies, including those on dreams.

(2) She did not particularly criticize Freud's dream theory. She actually followed his technique of dream interpretation without modification. However, in actual clinical practice, she gradually and implicitly adopted her own unique perspectives and methods of understanding dreams, although she did not state so clearly.

(3) In early analysis, Klein analysed the play of very young children by applying the technique of dream analysis there. She then discovered a world of object relation filled with sadistic fear in 0-year-old children. She applied dream analysis to examine children's play when they were awake, which led her to discover new analytical techniques and the psychology of 0-year-olds. In other words, she revealed important issues, including the fact that unconscious phantasy has an influence on children's play when they are awake, just like they have on dreams, and the fact that children's play expresses the internal object relations.

(4) Over time, in the treatment of adult manic-depression and adult schizophrenia, Klein began to consider that all free associations and actions when they were awake were influenced by and were ways to express their unconscious phantasies, similar to children's play. She also came to consider that dreams during sleep were manifestations of unconscious phantasies during sleep. She regarded here that, similar to children's play, adult's free associations themselves were expressions of unconscious phantasies. Accordingly, she developed a clinical technique to explore their unconscious meanings.

(5) Interpretation of adults' dreams: Klein used Freud's element association technique, without any modifications to treat adult patients. However, her understanding of the contents was greatly influenced by the theoretical viewpoints of the paranoid-schizoid position and depressive

position. That is, dreams were treated as an expression of the patients' internal state and unconscious phantasies of the early developmental stages. What she focused on there was early object relations, and she gave interpretations focusing on expressions of mental states such as persecutory anxiety, sadism, death instinct, depressive anxiety, and fear. The issues including late childhood Oedipal and sexual conflicts, which Freud paid attention to, has gradually lost importance.

(6) The theory of fulfilment of a wish was not emphasized much and became eclipsed. Simultaneously, anxiety dreams were not regarded as special, and they were treated equally as other dreams, merely as a sign of the patient's state of mind. Instead, Klein treated anxiety dreams and nightmares centrally as signs of early persecutory anxiety, fear of being abandoned, and depression.

(7) Terminology problems of interpretation: When Klein focused on the psychoanalysis of children, she used physical anatomical terms such as the mother's breast for children's play and dreams, and gave interpretations focusing on the destructive relationship with babies and the penis that exist inside the mother's physical body. However, after she began conducting adult psychoanalysis, she clarified the concept of the two positions. Subsequently, her focus changed to splitting, introjection, psychology of object loss, persecutory fear, and anxiety of annihilation, and her terms for interpretation also changed to adult functional terms.

4. Bion's perspective

Bion elucidated Klein's implicit modifications of Freud's method, and the conditions for having a dream:

(1) Dream thinking is important. During sleep, individuals turn their attention to the inner world, and the world of dream imagination is a place where the individuals' meaning of life arises. Additionally, passion is experience itself, and dreams are something that provides a formal expression to passion.

(2) The ability of an individual to dream is dependent on the activities of the non-psychotic part of his/her personality. There, the alpha function is active. It develops when infants can tolerate even when they are exposed to frustration and can retain their sensory impression without destroying it. It is fundamental to all mental activities, such as thinking, memorizing, dreaming, and imagining. When the psychotic part of an individual's personality is active, such as in schizophrenia, his/her ability to dream is also impaired.

(3) The function of the mother as a container also plays an important role in achieving this alpha function. In other words, when babies cannot endure their own experience, they attack their cognitive actions and sensory impressions, form fragmentations (beta elements), and project them onto their mothers. The containing ability of the mother to incorporate these elements and understand their meanings, and return them to the baby in an understandable and acceptable state for the baby is also an alpha effect. Then the mother converts the beta elements to alpha elements and returns them to the baby. After incorporating them, the baby can then use them as his/her own alpha elements. Simultaneously, the baby also incorporates the function of the mother's containment to enhance his/her alpha function. These conditions are important for the formation of the non-psychotic part of the personality, which is largely related to dream activities.

(4) Other proposals

(a) A dream, which is the development of an individual’s O, is an expression of a sensory experience. (b) A dream is a state of activity of unconscious phantasies during sleep. Unconscious phantasies are active in various forms, even when we are awake. (c) Dreams have the power to correct real frustration. (d) Emotional experiences are at the core of dreams. (e) Dreams are thoughts. (f) The manifestation of dreams is a chosen fact that resembles the state of the paranoid-schizoid position. (g) Bion gave dreams and thoughts an important mental position.

5. D. Meltzer's perspective

(1) Meltzer received direct guidance from Klein and conducted research as a child psychoanalyst. He believed that Klein also provided a new perspective on dream theory by advocating the theory of unconscious phantasy. Dreams do not occur as sleep guardians, although Freud said they did. Dreams are active both during sleep and when awake. They are called dreams if they occur during sleep and unconscious phantasies if they occur when the individual is awake.

(2) Such an inner world is where meaning occurs. It should be given an important role as 'dream life'.

6. Summary of H. Segal's perspective

Segal summarized opinions on dreams from a contemporary Kleinian perspective in an easy-to-understand manner.

(1) Dreams express unconscious phantasies, and the dream world is always with us, both during sleep and when awake.
(2) The language of dreams is very complex. This is related to what Freud considered as condensation, displacement, and symbolism.
(3) Dreams express compositions which form the personality, such as object relations, anxiety, and defence.
(4) Dream work is a complex process involving all related means of expression.
(5) The method of dream interpretation is the reverse process of dream work. In involves expanding a condensed dream, restoring the displacement to its original state, and breaking the code using element associations.

7. D. Fairbairn's perspective

Thus far, I have discussed the perspectives of Kleinian analysts. Here, I would like to introduce the theories and techniques concerning dreams proposed by the researchers of the independent group. In the UK, Kleinians and the researchers of the independent group have always influenced each other, and while their perspectives on dream theory have much in common, they have been developmentally criticizing and elaborating each other's theories.

Fairbairn's theory of dreams, which was published in the 1940s, was very innovative. He proposed that

(1) Dreams express the state of the inner world.
(2) The people who appear in dreams express a part of the dreamer's self.

In fact, he uses dreams as data about the individuals' internal correct answer. Using a patient's dream as an example, he proposed his famous structure of object relational personality. According to him, the earlier relation of frustration in the relation with the mother and the relationship of the self with the frustrating mother are unconsciously incorporated to form the personality structure. He considered dreams as expressions of such a state of personality. His idea of dreams that express the inner state has become one of the basic viewpoints of Kleinians and the object relation theorists.

8. C. Rycroft's perspective

Rycroft was the most active proponents of the role of dreams in contemporary object relations. His perspective had a significant influence on Kleinians and vice versa (1979). He proposed as follows:

(1) Although Freud proposed the theory of fulfilment of a wish, he ignored creative activities, and therefore, he regarded dreams as pathological. However, dreams should be considered as imaginary activities that occur during sleep. Imaginary activities are universal and they take place both during sleep and when awake. If an individual has a neurotic conflict, both dreams and imaginary activities that occur when he/she is awake are neurotic.
(2) There are two types of dreams: one is a 'fantastic dream', which simply expresses the inner world, and the other is an 'imaginative dream', which is filled with creative worlds.
(3) A dream means something and is a message to the dreamer.
(4) Dreams are very personal conversations. Therefore, they do not require general languages. Dreams are like videos because people mutually exchange special images in a non-arguing space. There is no need to express personal meanings universally there.

9. D. Winnicott's perspective

Winnicott said that dreaming itself has a meaning of play in the intermediate area and he emphasized the experience in the individual space when the patient tells the therapist that he/she had a dream.

As described earlier, current Kleinians regard the activity of dreams as the activity of unconscious phantasies, and consider dreams to be a form of expression when the individual is asleep, which convey his/her internal states. They try to understand the meaning of dreams by focusing on early object relations. They modified Freud's theoretical aspects by modifying Freud's developmental theory, but they carefully retained the importance of dream interpretation and techniques such as element analysis. They also emphasized the interpretation of transferences that appeared in dreams. Accordingly, they engaged in dream interpretation by considering not only the content of the dream but also the whole situation when the dream was recounted. The theoretical considerations of the researchers in the independent group also have a lot in common with those of Kleinians. There is an impression that they were conducting expansive research activities together. One other analyst who studied dreams was E. Sharpe. Her book is based on Freud's dream interpretation and its theory.

10. Case report

Here, I will introduce a case of clinical practice of dream interpretation in a part of the treatment of everyday analysis (50 minutes, 5 times a week). The patient was a married male patient Mr. A, who was in his 30s. His chief complaints included anthrophobia, lack of confidence in his profession, and lack of confidence as a husband and father.

He reported many dreams and showed significant self-understanding through the interpretation of dreams. Here, I would like to describe sessions from a week in which Mr. A reported many dreams, after about a year from the start of treatment. The description mainly relates to the analysis of dreams, but it also shows the importance of transference interpretation in dream analysis and the forms of resistance of dreams. Due to space limitations, free associations about the dream elements are omitted, except for the necessary sections.

(1) Monday

Mr. A mentioned a mistake he had made in the previous week. He mistakenly said that his male cousin's house, in which Mr. A lived together with him for a while, was dirty, instead of saying that his cousin's feet were dirty. He then stated that, since childhood, his cousin's life was full of deprived experiences and that his cousin was abandoned by his parents. He said that his cousin was too harsh and difficult. Mr. A thought that he was released when his cousin went on a trip for a while. He said that he could have a safe sex life with no worries, and he said he suddenly masturbated early in the morning. He then reported a dream: "I met three very angry women. The last girl was pretty, but later, I found out that she was my acquaintance's daughter." This acquaintance had ruined his own family by gambling. The therapist asked Mr. A if he felt that he was making a big bet by changing jobs. Mr. A said that he was borrowing money from his cousin and that he felt sorry about it. Additionally, Mr. A had borrowed money from his own father too, and he felt extremely guilty about it. Mr. A then said that a man, who had also changed jobs, was very upset that he could no longer return to his hometown, and wondered whether the man had rung the bell of the therapist's office. The therapist interpreted that the man also represented Mr. A himself, and that it indicated that he was extremely upset. The therapist also interpreted that the three angry women represented Mr. A's wife, his mother-in law, and his own mother.

(2) Tuesday

Mr. A described his feeling of self-condemnation that it was as if he was stealing money from his cousin and father. The therapist interpreted that Mr. A felt that he was stealing something from the therapist. Mr. A was worried because he did not know what kind of job he could get. He then reported the following dream: "I was in a certain country and spying. I knew there was a factory that made new weapons. I had to find out where it was. I found a secret entrance, and went underground to the bottom. I knew the factory was nearby. It was a station that I knew well. Then the scene changed suddenly. I was with a famous novelist and movie director. We were looking at a beautiful building, but that was my house or my grandmother's house. We praised the architect's skills. The roof was covered with artificial snow, which could not be distinguished from natural snow. I was sorry that the house was to be burned at the end of the movie. I then went home with my childhood friend, with our arms around each other's shoulders." After the element associations, the therapist gave interpretations that Mr. A was trying to spy on the therapist's mind, and that he felt that the therapist had a weapon that would severely destroy Mr. A's mind. On the other hand, the two famous figures represented the therapist and Mr. A, and Mr. A felt that they were creating a wonderful piece of work together. The beautiful house probably represented the therapist's and A's own ability to understand, which will collapse at the end of the session. Additionally, Mr. A said that the background in the dream resembled the scenery he had seen when he visited his wife's parents' house, and recalled the time when he visited his wife's parents to ask them to allow him to marry their daughter. Furthermore, Mr. A recalled that there was a building of his hometown among the houses of an analyst. The therapist interpreted that Mr. A was trying to obtain something so important in his life during treatment, and that his intention was to penetrate into the therapist to build a beautiful building of his hometown, which represented his strength. There was a phase here in which the boundary between the therapist and Mr. A became unclear, and the creativity and ability of the therapist, the ability acquired by the patient, and the ability he originally possessed were mixed up. This shows that Mr. A's idealization, identification, and envy towards the therapist were extremely strong.

(3) Wednesday

Mr. A first mentioned that his colleague injured his arm and was wearing a bandage. The colleague was also receiving psychoanalytic treatment from the same therapist as Mr. A. Mr. A felt that his colleague was getting along better with the therapist. Thus, he thought that the colleague got his arm injured because he felt guilty towards Mr. A. Then, Mr. A reported the following dream: "I was in a lab where the therapist was hypnotizing a stupid man. He was a man who worked in my workplace. The man turned into a baby and rolled on the floor and cried. I was surprised at the therapist's ability to control people's mind. When I was looking at books on the bookshelf, I noticed that one of the bookshelves was a secret door. There was an evacuation port with a grip bar that could be used in case of an emergency fire. The therapist came from the next room and fell from there. I thought the therapist injured his head." The other dream was as follows: "I was attending a workshop where a versatile man was giving a presentation. He seemed to have been a champion of something when he was young, and later he wrote a book on Shakespeare and was also a talented painter. The man's face resembled the face of a clerk at the workplace where I once worked. When I went home, the road was a country road. I told my neighbourhood classmate that my horse was tired, and I asked him to give me a ride on his back. He accepted and put me on his back, but on the way home my classmate kissed me, and I was thrown into confusion." As for the first dream, Mr. A talked about the Jewish girl Anne Frank. She was hiding with her family behind a camouflaged door. Mr. A stated a feeling of emptiness about the hole. He said that the neighbourhood man was once a gentle man, but after he grew into an adult, he became terribly aggressive. As for the man in his workplace, Mr. A said he was extremely discouraged about him. This was because, one day, the man said that he could not understand Mr. A at all. Additionally, Mr. A spoke of his chief, who criticized him very harshly in front of a customer.

Mr. A's first dream, which expressed the dominant power of the therapist, represented his competitiveness and jealousy against his colleague (who was a patient of the same therapist). The therapist interpreted that Mr. A felt that his colleague was receiving special treatment, and that he wished his colleague would get hurt and that the treatment would fall into a terrible state. Then, the therapist was found and murdered, just like Anne Frank's family. Mr. A wished that such a dominant therapist, who favours one patient over another, should also be murdered. The talented man also represented his colleague patient and also a part of the therapist. Mr. A was jealous of the abilities of his colleague and therapist. Furthermore, when the therapist had even the slightest difficulty in understanding Mr. A, Mr. A felt disappointed and disrespected the therapist. In such situations, Mr. A wanted to speak ill about the therapist publicly. When the therapist was unreliable, Mr. A wanted to rely on another therapist. However, he then shivered with homosexual fear. The empty hole represented the anus, which expressed a homosexual disposition. As for the fire, Mr. A gave an association of burning the house of the movie set at the end of the movie in the dream he had the day before. The therapist interpreted that it was related to separation before a vacation, and that it was related to anger that would burn everything out.

(4) Thursday

The first dream was as follows: "A junior high school teacher was riding a horse in a muddy field. The horse could not move forward smoothly and it went backwards sometimes. However, the teacher managed the horse well and was having fun. I was moving along a narrow path in the bushes, and then, another teacher got on a horse." The second dream was as follows: "I was with my wife and daughter. My daughter went to take ballet lessons. My wife insisted that our daughter should come home alone because it would make her independent. I thought that it would be worrisome."

The therapist interpreted that, "The horses represent the father's and the therapist's penis and abilities, and they can use them well. Mr. A is envious of them." Mr. A told the therapist that his father brought a wasteland under cultivation and his mother planted pasture grass there. The therapist interpreted that this represents Mr. A's parents' sexual intercourse, and it was a creative story about having children. Mr. A had felt that the therapeutic experience was creating something new through collaboration (sexual intercourse) with the therapist. Mr. A gave an association of the story of the "Blue Horse". In the story, a child's mother died, and he lived with his father. On one occasion, the boy met a blue horse. They became friends and the horse carried the boy very quickly. The horse told the boy that he must not tell anyone about that. One day, the boy's father suddenly became ill. The boy called his horse and went to call a doctor. Thanks to the horse, his father was saved. The boy unintentionally told his father about the horse. Since that day, the blue horse disappeared. That night, the boy had a dream of his mother. His mother's eyes were same as the eyes of the blue horse. The therapist stated that this was an indication of Mr. A's inseparability from the therapist and that it was related to the separation experience before a vacation. The therapist further interpreted that the blue horse represented masturbation, which caused the father to become sick. However, Mr. A was put off by this interpretation. Then, Mr. A gave an association on his son. His son was sick but he recovered and wanted to learn everything. His son wanted the same things as his younger brother and became very twisted. The therapist interpreted that Mr. A did not want to listen to what the therapist told him and was concerned that the therapist might make Mr. A go home alone, as in the dream, or tell him to discontinue treatment. The therapist interpreted that this was deeply related with the vacation.

(5) Friday

Mr. A stated that he did not understand exactly why the previous day's dream had to do with masturbation, and he was put off by the idea. He then said that he had an uninteresting dream again.

The first dream was as follows: "I live in a house in a wooded area at the top of a mountain. A man whom I knew, Mr. T, visited me. Mr. T is a completely henpecked husband. We both went somewhere, but suddenly I was holding two babies. I became Mr. T, and held one of the babies. Mr. T was dumped by the woman he liked. There were rumours that she liked me instead." The second dream was as follows: "I was looking at a man who was hang gliding. He was about to take off from the school ground, but the hang glider turned into a toy airplane. It flew very well and could hover in the air. If we did not hide, we would have been shot with machine guns." Then, Mr. A talked about his colleague who was having an affair and said that he felt jealous of him. He further said that, in the dream, a man said he wanted to marry his wife.

Mr. A said that these dreams were confusing and that he did not know what he was saying. He also said that he was confused because the therapist talked about his parents' sexual intercourse. As for the hang glider, Mr. A wanted to hang glide when he was young, but he could not because he was afraid of a crash. He also wanted to be an airplane designer when he was a child. The therapist said that they represented the patient's penis and that mastering a profession was also his attempt to gain the power of a penis. Mr. A further talked about a friend who visited him, saying that he was highly educated but could not speak English and that his daughter had abandoned home and gone abroad. The therapist had to end the treatment without fully understanding the meaning of these dreams because the time had come. Here, perhaps the dreams themselves were used for resistance of treatment, and were thought to represent confusion and protest against the therapist's misinterpretation (probably the interpretation of the blue horse); however, the therapist did not have a chance to point it out until the end.

11. Considerations

As seen above, patients report many dreams in everyday analysis, and the transference analyses of these dreams often bring important developments. In the work where patients have dreams and report them, and the therapist who listened to them shows an understanding, there exists an important therapeutic process which was pointed out by the Kleinians and the object relation theorists mentioned earlier. The therapist fundamentally approaches the patients with the basic techniques of dream analysis. What is most characteristic about the approach is that the therapist gives interpretations focusing on the internal situation in early object relation and its transference relation. Moreover, anatomical interpretation terms are not used often, and interpretations are based on using everyday functional words.

It was evident from this case that, while being surprised with his own creativity, the patient scrutinized the therapist's interpretation of the dreams, and expanded his self-understanding. However, on the other hand, his dreams clearly showed feelings of jealousy and envy against the therapist's ability, as well as suspicions and criticism of the invalidity of the therapist's interpretations. Additionally, the patient had too many dreams and provided too many associations for the therapist to understand them all. By doing so, the patient attempted to prevent further progress of self-understanding through dreams, or tried to hinder the therapist's unsatisfactory interpretations. Therefore, it is important to take into account not only just the content of the dreams but also how patients use dreams to resist.

12. Conclusion

This paper introduced the development of dream theory and dream interpretation techniques since Freud, focusing on the work of Kleinians and object-relations theorists. Additionally, I attempted to demonstrate the importance of dream interpretation in everyday analysis by presenting a case report in which the patient recounted abundant dreams.

References

1) Bion, Wilfred Ruprecht. 1962. *Learning from Experience*. London: Heinemann.
2) Bion, Wilfred Ruprecht. 1963. *The Elements of Psychoanalysis*. London: Heinemann.
3) Bion, Wilfred Ruprecht. 1965. *Transformation*. London: Heinemann.
4) Bion, Wilfred Ruprecht. 1970/1977. *Attention and Interpretation*. London: Heinemann.
5) Fairbairn, Donald. 1952. *Psychoanalytic Studies of the Personality*. London: Routledge.
6) Freud, Sigmund. 1900. "Interpretation of Dreams". In *Standard Edition*, Vol. 4-5. London: Hogarth Press.
7) Kinugasa, Takayuki. 1991. "Dream Theory in Object Relation". *Imago*, Extra Edition "Dreams", Vol. 2-12 (in Japanese)
8) Kinugasa, Takayuki. 1997 "Analysis of Dreams: Development from

Klein to Bion". *L'esprit d'aujourd'hui*, Extra Issue "Analysis of dreams" (in Japanese)
9) Klein, Melanie. 1984. *The Writings of Melanie Klein*, Vol. 1-3. London: Hogarth Press.
10) Meltzer, Donald. 1984. *Dream-Life*. London: Clunie Press.
11) Rycroft, Charles. 1979. *The Innocence of Dreams*. London: Hogarth Press.
12) Segal, Hanna. 1991. *Dream, Phantasy and Art*. London: Routledge.
13) Sharpe, Ella. 1937. *Dream Analysis*. London: Hogarth Press.
14) Winnicott, Donald Woods. 1971. *Playing and Reality*. London: Routledge.

[1998. *The Japanese Journal of Psycho-analysis*, Vol. 42, No. 3.]

ON FREUD'S CASES

CHAPTER 16

THERAPEUTIC FACTORS FOR THE RAT MAN IN VIEW OF OBJECT RELATION

1. Introduction

Among Freud's cases, the Rat Man case is special in several respects.

First, this is the only case Freud left a record of the first four months of therapy. The records were discovered after his death and was published in English by Lytton Strachey in 1954. Since Freud had a habit of discarding his patient records, this case is a valuable material for understanding the actuals of his routine clinical practice. By referring to both Freud's published papers and clinical records on Rat Man, the facts of his theoretical thinking and clinical techniques are easier to study than other cases.

It seems that he concentrated his effort the most on this case. This is because his "identification" with this patient can be strongly seen. For example, he accidentally recorded the patient's lover with his ex-lover's name, Gisela Fluss, and identification is expressed from the fact that Freud himself put an exclamation mark after the name.

On the other hand, despite Freud's such great enthusiasm and interest, treatment lasted only 11 months (9 and a half months according to Mahony P. J.). However, the patient was relieved of obsessive-compulsive symptoms, managed to do his job, and two years later, and married his long-cherished lover. Unfortunately, he later died in World War I.

By the way, when considering Freud's cases, there are always specific problems. When criticizing case studies of the founder of psychoanalysis, we psychoanalysts have some special hesitation. It is also difficult to understand the meaning of the case unless Freud's own developmental revision of techniques and theories are taken into account. Many researchers have addressed various points and criticisms for Freud's case, but it is hard to provide a viewpoint comparable to those points. Furthermore, critics become quite defensive since they become concerned that what they were going to say maybe something that someone has already pointed out.

2. Characteristics of the case

There are many excellent studies regarding clinical consideration for this case and the major characteristics include the followings. These become the basic background when considering this case.

(1) This case became the centre of Freud's research on obsessional neurosis.
(2) The focus is on the pathology of object loss with respect to the death of Rat Man's father.
(3) Although clinical records mention Rat Man's relationships with women, such as his mother and his lover, as much as with his father, Freud rarely took them up in his published papers.
(4) Unlike the Dora case, Freud did not positively give dream interpretations.
(5) Symptoms consist of complex compulsive acts and ideas. They are often erotized in treatment and Freud tends to get involved in the world. However, at this point, Freud's therapeutic goal was to reveal the developmental experiences and memories of early childhood regarding symptom formation.
(6) In the first seven sessions, Freud gave Rat Man many intellectual lectures on phenomena such as resistance and unconsciousness. These lectures might have served also as diagnostic interviews and introductory interviews, but there is a possibility that Freud gave more intellectual lectures to Rat Man than to other cases because he had particular interest in this case.
(7) The free association method may not have been the completed version of his latter period.
(8) The concept of transferences during this period was in transition and had not evolved much from the meaning discovered from the Dora case. Transferences were used as a means of recalling hidden memories, not as here-and-now, and were not used as a relationship with the therapist. Additionally, when Freud refers to transferences, they are emotions or ideas which the patient consciously directs to the therapist. Freud did not mention unconscious transferences.
(9) Interpretations consist mostly of genetic reconstructions. The transference relationship with the therapist was hardly interpreted. It can be considered that Freud did not yet have a clear view on its importance at this point.

(10) The therapeutic goal was to assist the patient to become aware of his unconscious idea that he brought about the cause of his father's death.

(11) Freud had a keen interest in clarifying the formation process of obsessive-compulsive symptoms and their unconscious meanings as a pathological study. This was a tendency that can been seen from Freud's "Studies on Hysteria". At this point, becoming conscious of the transference relationships, which is the new therapeutic goal, was not clarified.

(12) At this point, Freud had no clear view on the therapeutic significance of counter-transferences.

3. More specific problems

The specific problems are related to counter-transferences and technical issues and they are associated to Freud's behaviour which deviated quite far beyond the principle of the "therapist's neutrality", which Freud proposed later. His clinical records include the following matters:

(1) At an early stage, Freud requested a photo of the patient's lover.
(2) Freud gave the patient a book which fit the patient's theme.
(3) Freud offered the patient a meal.
(4) Freud sent the patient a summer greeting card.
(5) Freud inquired to the patient's mother about the circumstances where the patient was severely chastised by his father.
(6) The patient came to Freud's clinic to provide assistance to an epileptic patient. (However, the facts about this are not clear.)

The patient experienced these acts as intrusive approaches from Freud. In particular, offering a meal before the treatment time is an act that cannot be understood in the common sense of current psychoanalysis. The patient experienced this that he was given oral stimuli and developed sexual and persecutory phantasies. Freud did not seem to particularly have an awareness of the problems involved.

4. Problem of counter-transferences

Freud had a life experience similar to that of the patient, which is said to have enhanced Freud's identification with the patient (Mahony). The patient was born when his father was 53 years old, and his mother was 19 years younger than his father. These are very similar to the ages of Freud's parents.

The patient's relationship with his father was reminiscent of Freud's relationship with his father. The patient's hometown was near the hometown of Freud's family, and the patient was Jewish and had to move to Vienna to start a new life, just like Freud's family.

Both the patient and Freud had lost their elder sisters at an early age. The patient is also a medical student (Recently it is said that he was a lawyer). In addition, regarding his marriage, the patient was trying to marry his cousin, whom his parents did not hope for, breaking the family conventions and expectations. Moreover, his lover's name was Gisela, the same name of the woman who was Freud's first love. When Freud married his wife Marta, he fought against Jewish customs and won the marriage, but he had experienced a conflict that it might have been better to marry a woman born in a wealthy family like his cousin (niece), and become a business person, as his father wanted him to be. These factors are said to have promoted Freud's counter-transferences. As Mahony says, Freud's writings give a particularly warm and empathetic impression towards Rat Man compared to the cases of Dora and Wolfman.

As mentioned above, at this point, Freud had not yet had a clear awareness regarding the therapeutic significance and importance of counter-transference.

5. Therapeutic factors from the viewpoint of object relation

The object relation theory originated in Klein's theory, and in particular, the theories of the "paranoid-schizoid position" and the "depressive position" in the latter half of her research life are one of the most representative theories in object relations theory. I, the author, would like to make an object relation-theoretic consideration in this perspective.

According to Klein's theory on neurosis, when "depressive anxiety" in the "depressive position", which includes the anxiety of losing the object, the feeling of guilt for attacking the object, the anxiety of destructing the object by attacking it, and the feeling of object-seeking, cannot be dealt only by primitive defences, it is considered that neurotic mechanisms are used without the patient regressing into the world of the "paranoid-schizoid position" because the ego has a certain degree of strength. Obsessive-compulsive symptoms are one of the mechanisms, and basically, they come to present the problem of ambivalence with the object in the "depressive position". There, a situation occurs where the ambivalence with the patient's mother, the primary object, the dyadic relational conflict with his father, the conflict with his siblings centring on love and hatred with their parents, the early Oedipal complex and the early super-ego are intricately intertwined. The therapeutic goal is to work-through each of the patient's ambivalent conflicts with these objects, and this is conducted through transferences.

As for the problems in the later stages of the "depressive position", the object appears as a whole object, so in order to highlight the object-relational perspective, I would like to focus on the patient's ambivalent relationship with his subjective mother image and father image, and the characteristics of the maternal transferences to Freud.

(1) Pathology of object loss for his father's death

What Freud viewed the most important in this case was the patient's conflict over his father, who died nine years ago. The patient suffered badly before his father's death from guilt hoping for his father to die, and he had been in pain because he fell asleep and could not be by his father's deathbed. In addition, after he developed obsessive-compulsive symptoms, he was haunted with the phantasy that his father would come back at the same time of his death. He suffered from a strong obsessive idea to harm his father and his loved one, who would not accept him, with the rat torture, which he heard from his military boss, and tried to counteract it with complex compulsive acts and magical omnipotence.

It seems that the patient's tendency to "introject" and "identify" with his father was enhanced during his experience in the military. He experienced a strong conflict between the feeling that he should abandon his poor lover and get married to a wealthy woman, just as his father did, and the fact that his actual lover Gisela was a sick and infertile woman who was neither from a good family nor rich. The father was the closest person to the patient. Just as his father and mother were cousins, Rat Man also selected his cousin as his object.

However, his father was a womaniser, a gambler, and a prodigal. That tendency seemed to have been particularly strong while his father was in the military. Freud considered that the anecdote that when the patient's father lost all his money in gambling, he could not finally pay back the debt to a colleague who kindly paid the money for him was related to the obsessive-compulsive symptoms of the patient who strongly "identified" with his father.

There is a possibility that his father had left large debts. According to the patient, his father was also a low-born, uncultivated, and vulgar person. The patient was critical of such a father, but in reality, the patient had also "introjected" such father, and gambled, was sexually unrestrained seducing many women and wasting money limitlessly on women. He also suffered from the guilt of possessing fierce aggression and hoping his death against his father, who severely tortured him and his younger sister. However, the patient himself, like his father, would spasmodically attack his younger sister and other women.

For these reasons, Freud believed that the patient's suffering from responsibility for the death of his father was at the core of the patient's pathology.

Freud also thought that the patient's inability to handle the "mourning work" of his father's death well was related to the problem of his older sister, who died when the patient was little.

Freud's attention on the conflicts between the guilt and aggression regarding the failure of "mourning work" for the bereavement of the father, and the patient's "introjection" of his father after the bereavement are highly object-relational perspectives. However, the characteristic of Freud's work is that he focused concentratively on the conflict with his father.

(2) Ambivalent internal relationship with his mother

The mother was always retreated in the background for Freud's pathology. Like other cases such as the Dora case, Hans case, Schreber case, and Wolfman case, a pathology centred on the father is developed in the consideration of this case. However, in Freud's four-month detailed clinical records based on his clinical observing eye, the patient referred to his mother as much as to his father, especially in the latter half.

According to the clinical record, the patient's mother was the ruler of the family, and it was the mother who actually wanted to marry a wealthy man of good birth. It was the mother who felt she has failed by marrying a man without money. The mother had always lamented to the patient about her husband's issues including gambling and there is a possibility that she complained to the patient that he should never marry a wealthless woman or be like his father.

It seems that the mother herself was an adopted child and had an early deprivation experience, and her adoptive father treated her adoptive mother harshly, so she grew up in an unfortunate environment at home. Accordingly, she had a nagging, fastidious and stingy personality, which may be the result of "identification" with her adoptive father.

The patient had unconscious anger toward such mother, and, there is a possibility that he introjected the part of the prodigal father, which his mother disliked the most, to rebel against her by sympathizing and identifying with his father. It can also be considered that he chose Gisela, a wealthless woman who could not give birth to a child, with a retaliatory intention to shatter such mother's expectation. However, when he first confessed his love to Gisela (two years before his father's death), a woman who urged him to love her committed suicide around the same time. The mother bitterly complained to the patient about this, and it can be assumed that she admonished him for his prodigality analogous to his father's.

The patient may have believed that the father's indulgence in gambling was due to his mother's regret for marrying a man who was not from a good family nor had any wealth, or for her insidious accusations and attacks. He may have sympathized with his father. Identifying with such a part of his father would have been the most powerful rebellion against his mother.

(3) Maternal transference to Freud and identification with his mother

Freud focused his interest on the father problem thus was somewhat confused when the maternal transferences to Freud began to develop. Since the conflict between the patient and his father was important to Freud as the core of the pathology, while the patient talked about his conflict with his mother, it seems that Freud just recorded what could not be integrated by his theory and what he observed as they were.

It is not clear why Freud did not keep the clinical records after the fourth month (or maybe he just happened to lose them), but after the records broke off, the aggressive relationship between the patient and his mother became more prominent. It may be because the patient's mother complained to Freud or told him that she would make the patient discontinue treatment. Or, since the emotions of maternal transference to Freud became stronger, many phenomena which Freud could not explain by the father conflict theory may have begun to emerge, and Freud could not handle them.

I would like to return to the clinical records, and give a consideration focusing on the last two months of them. The last two months is from late November 1907, when the patient clearly began to have various transference fantasies to Freud and dreams and expressly state his relationship with his mother, up to mid-January 1908, when the clinical records broke off. The main theme of this part of the clinical records focuses on the patient's transference relationship with his mother and Freud.

While talking about his issues such as neurosis on the relationship with his lover, the patient suddenly began reporting various fantasies and dreams for Freud and his family from November 21, 1907. This lasted about 20 days until December 10.

The images for Freud's daughter were a fantasy of her doing a fellatio for the patient and him licking her, and a dream having anal sex with her back-to-back through faeces. Later, the patient had a dream where Freud's daughter had lumps of "poop" on each of her eyes. Freud considered these were paternal transferences and associated them with the patient's question of whether to marry the wealthy Freud's daughter or his own lover.

However, I think they have yet another meaning. They mean that the patient treated other women crudely only as objects of sexuality, just in the same way as his mother despised young women who did not come from good families. In that sense, here the patient was "identified" with his arrogant and proud mother.

In addition, the patient held a conviction that a relative of Freud was the murderer of the train murder case, expressing his suspicion and underestimation against and fear of being retaliated by Freud with aggression and criminality. The patient gave an association that among his relatives, there was an uncle who fled the country for fraud, which here rather implies his father transference.

The patient also has the following dreams. "Freud's mother was stabbed in her breast with a Japanese sword and her genitals were eaten by Freud and her other children." "Freud's mother is dead. I wonder if I should I tell my condolences. I might burst out laughing." "Freud's mother was in despair because all her children had been hung by the neck and were dead." These were probably the patient's expressions of aggression towards his mother which the patient presented as Freud's experiences, using the mechanism of "projective identification" to Freud. There are themes where the patient destroys his mother's breasts, eats genitals, commits murder, and kills other children of his mother. This is a manifestation of the sadism in the early object relation with the mother, which Klein described in the papers on psychoanalysis for the children.

Moreover, the patient had a dream where there was a dead child sleeping in-between Freud and his wife. This indicated the patient's jealousy for Freud's child, and also the patient's possessiveness toward Freud. It may also be an expression of his Oedipal complex to his parents. Touching the primal scene of his parents means death for the patient. (This will be stated below.)

At the end of a series of transference fantasies, the patient had the following dream. "Several children were lying down, and Freud's child was there, too. I was giving something to them. It was brown and wonderful. The children were licking what was around their mouths. In the end, Freud gives it to his mother." Freud associated this dream to the episode where the patient's younger brother ate faeces when he was little. Freud seemed to have thought this was an expression of the patient's aggression, where the patient made the children and even the mother eat faeces. Of course, thorough aggression, underestimation, and destruction against the good things the patient gave and received are seen here, but probably it also represents an aspect of the patient's good experience with Freud. In return, the patient identified his self to Freud and became an existence that gave good food to others. The dream also seems to express the phantasy of giving something good to his mother.

Around this time, the patient reported that his mother was an adopted child and that her adoptive father was ruthless. The patient then began to behave arrogantly and harshly to Freud, like his own mother, and began to condemn Freud for minute things. The patient said Freud had bad manners and refused to shake hands with him saying he was filthy because he would pick his nose. In regard to this, Freud correctly stated that the patient was "identifying" with his mother. However, Freud did not address the issue of ambivalence for the mother as a pathology for obsessional neurosis. He stated that it was difficult to find an association between rats and the patient's mother.

From mid-December, the patient no longer had any aggressions or transference fantasies for Freud, and Freud stated that the transferences had disappeared. The patient suddenly began attacking and condemning his mother. He detested the smell of his mother's genitals and began to directly vent his anger on her. He also stated that he inherited all his bad aspects from his mother. The patient also acted as if he were his mother and began to say ridiculous things all day long like her. That is, he opposed everything his younger sister did and began to criticize his lover's cousin and his aunt. In addition, he criticized Freud that he did not understand anything, and began to complain about his father in the same way as his mother. He then had a dream of "his mother denouncing his father for returning home after a long absence".

In this way, the patient repeatedly attacked his mother directly or Freud, who was the object of maternal transference, or conversely "identified with" his mother and attacked Freud and other family members. This is probably a manifestation of the patient's unresolved ambivalent conflict towards his mother.

The problematic "meal" incidence occurred on December 28, 1907. In the same session, Freud gave the patient a novel written by Zora which dealt with the same theme as the patient.

The following day, the patient had the following dream about this. "Freud's wife and his mother were connected though a herring sticking out from their anuses. A girl cut it in two." Freud does not specifically give an interpretation on this. There was actually a herring in the patient's meal of the day before. The patient disliked herrings and left it all. It seems to express the patient's rejection and underestimation of the most maternal thing the therapist gave him, that is food. In other words, what he was given was the same as faeces, which was made by a woman in Freud's family from her anus. This can be considered to be "identification" with the mother (=

grandfather) and also aggression against the mother (= grandmother). The patient demeaned and rejected, like his mother, what Freud's family gave to him, while on the other hand, projected his mother and grandmother who fed him to Freud's family and attacked the good mother-grandmother image trying to destroy it. In this respect, it can be said that the patient was also identified with his harsh grandfather. The patient's grandfather treated his grandmother ruthlessly, and his mother was probably identified with his grandfather. The patient later denounced and slandered Freud's interpretation, stating that Freud sought to benefit from giving him a meal.

He then had the following dream. "The dentist accidentally pulled out a tooth that didn't hurt." [(1) (6) (7)] Although Freud associated this with the death of a patient's relative, considering from the context, it would be more appropriate to think that the patient was conveying that Freud was pursuing the wrong theme. In any case, Freud at that time rarely gave here-and-now dream interpretations.

As described above, the patient rapidly went through transitions including paternal transference, maternal transference, and "identification" with his mother using mechanisms such as "projection" and "projective identification".

(4) Characteristics of the Oedipal complex

As mentioned above, the patient's father was a useless person castrated by the patient's mother. However, when he had a tantrum, he was also a father who also punished the patient severely. He was a man who has no assets and married being blinded by money. He was a prodigal gambling father who died leaving debts. However, he was also a close beloved father for the patient.

The patient's mother was a prideful, nagging, aggressive woman obsessive with cleanliness. She always controlled the patient, and insisted that he must not be like his father, and that he should marry a rich woman. She probably did not get along well with her husband, and her husband often would be away from their house.

For the patient, such a parental relationship was a composition in which his strong mother controlled and castrated his father. Nevertheless, for the phantasy where his parents had a special intimate relationship and he was excluded, there is a possibility that the patient directed an image of destructive parents and had a primal scene phantasy where they destroyed and dirtied each other as in the anal stage (anal stage Oedipal complex). Such combination of the parents is not creative but becomes a hotbed for aggression and destructiveness. Infants develop a severe early superego to guarantee the compensatory false self and develop a personality that is prone to feel strong guilt. This has appeared in the patient's intense guilt when the father died and his Oedipal desire was fulfilled (e.g., the fantasy that if the father died, he can marry his lover [mother's deputy]) and in his intense "introjection" in object loss when he lost his dyadic relational beloved father. (Freud did not give a detailed consideration on Oedipal complex in this case.)

Furthermore, the patient "identified" with his castrating mother, accusing his father of being a prodigal, and may have thought that it would be better if his father disappeared. (This is also a form of the destructive early Oedipus complex). When his father actually died, the feeling of guilt that he had inadvertently destroyed his beloved father, and the restitution desire by introjecting his father may have been enhanced.

(5) Object relational therapeutic factors

As Mahony states, it is likely that the improvement of Rat Man's symptoms was a transference cure. However, it can also be said that Freud's decisive seeking for the pathology of conflict over the patient's loss experience of his father, which considerably resolved the problems, greatly contributed to the disappearance of the symptoms. Moreover, the patient may have obtained an opportunity of a strong "identification" as Freud perpetually pursued the developmental causal relationship of the meaning of symptom formation.

In object relation theory, it is considered that, as for the cases of neurosis, resolving the pathology of the "depressive position" in transferences is a therapeutically important factor. Therapy consisted of solving the therapeutic transferences of the ambivalent relationship with the pre-Oedipus mother, and also of the dyadic relational conflict with the father through here-and-now interpretations; and interpreting the manifestations of the various stages of activities of the early Oedipal complex, which is assumed to start around 6 months from birth, and the super-ego.

From this point of view, in the Rat Man case, the ambivalent relationship with the pre-Oedipus mother emerged from about the second month of treatment through transferences and entered the stage where it was necessary to interpret this relationship. Although it is unknown to what extent this was conducted since there are no records, as mentioned above, treatment for this patient was ended relatively early. There is a possibility that therapy was finally discontinued in response to the mother's pressure because the patient's intense acting-out was induced without the maternal transferences and the conflict with the patient's actual mother being adequately interpreted.

In any case, it can be considered that the patient's experience of turning his hatred and aggression for his mother through transferences to Freud or directly to her worked to reduce the patient's conflict, although Freud did not positively interpret it.

(6) Freud's dream interpretation

In this case, Freud was not as positive about dream interpretation as in the Dora case. He stated that academic interest must be sacrificed for the treatment of patients. Perhaps he said so because he reflected that he was too driven by his academic interest in dream interpretation in the Dora case.

In fact, Rat Man reported many noteworthy dreams, and it is very interesting to interpret them anew. However, I would like to save this for another time due to space limitations.

(7) Obsession of the rat torture

Freud gave considerations on the patient's various obsessive-compulsive symptoms and their relationship with his father's gambling and debts, babies, and penis in line with the origins of the patient's psychic development.

On the other hand, in view of the aggression against the nagging and dominant mother who repeated slander, it can be inferred that the rat is the patient himself. The rat (Rat Man), who was trapped (in the world controlled by his mother) and had his escape cut off, had a fantasy of causing (his mother's) death by entering the body from an anus or female genitals and biting off internal organs. It's appearance as an obsessive idea while giving the patient so much fear and anxiety seems to be related to the fact that he possessed aggression and destructiveness toward his mother. This seems to be a symbolism of the sadistic phantasies of the later oral stage and anal stage, in which babies bite off their mother's breast and inside of her body with their sharp teeth. This psychic activity, which was an introjection of partial objects, was carried out also in the same way for his father.

The patient's lover partially had the image of the patient's mother (Gisela lost her father at an early age and was sexually abused by her adoptive father, which is similar to the patient's mother's personal history). When Gisela rejected Rat Man, it meant for Rat Man that he was rejected by his mother and he would be taken into a world where he would be made to marry a wealthy woman in line with his mother's intentions. In that sense, the obsessive idea of conducting the rat torture to Gisela, who rejected him, may have been his aggression for his mother. Actually, the patient had a fantasy that Gisela would enter the body of a whore (her mother = Rat Man's mother) and have sexual intercourse with the patient, and then she would explode and his mother would come apart, too. Gisela was partly a mother to the patient and partly represented the world of the patient who rebelled against his mother's world. This may be one of the reasons why Rat Man's symptoms were exacerbated when he was rejected by Gisela.

6. Conclusion

As seen above, regarding the Rat Man case, I presented the accomplishments of previous researches and gave them historical positions. I then gave considerations focusing on the clinical records from an object relational perspective on the matters including the patient's maternal transference, mourning work related to the bereavement with his father and the anal-stage Oedipus complex. Dream analysis was omitted due to the limited number of papers. Furthermore, I considered the meaning of the rat torture obsession from the viewpoint of early mother-child relationship.

References

(1) Freud, Sigmund. 1909. "Notes Upon a Case of Obsessional Neurosis". In *Standard Edition*, Vol. 10: 155-320. London: Hogarth Press.

(2) Freud, Sigmund. 1954: "Addendum: Original Record of the Case". In *Standard Edition*, Vol. 10: 253-318. London: Hogarth Press.

(3) Gottlieb, Richard. M. 1989. "Technique and Countertransference in Freud's Analysis of the Rat Man". *Psychoanalytic Quarterly*, Vol. 58: 29-62.

(4) Kanzer, Mark, and Glenn, Jules, ed. 1980: *Freud and his Patients*. New York: Jason Aronson.

(5) Lipton, Samuel. 1977. "The Advantages of Freud's Technique as Shown in His Analysis of the Rat Man". *International Journal of Psychoanalysis*, Vol. 58: 255-73.

(6) Lipton, Samuel. 1979. "An Addendum to "The Advantages of Freud's Technique as Shown in His Analysis of the Rat Man"". *International Journal of Psychoanalysis*, Vol. 60: 215-16.

(7) Mahony, Patrick. J. 1986. *Freud and the Rat Man*. New Haven: Yale University Press.

(8) Muslin, Hyman L. 1979. "Transference in the Rat Man Case: The Transference in Transition". *Journal of the American Psychoanalytic Association*, Vol. 27: 561-577.

(9) Okonogi, Keigo. 1973. *Freud – Traces of the Ego, NHK Books*. Tokyo: NHK Publishing (in Japanese)

(10) Okonogi, Keigo. 1977. "Obsessional Neurosis seen Psychoanalytically – Freud and after". *The Japanese Journal of Psycho-analysis*, Vol. 21, No. 4: 163-179 (in Japanese)
(11) Okonogi, Keigo. 1979. *Object Loss -To Mourn-*. Tokyo: Chuokoron-Shinsha, Inc. (in Japanese)

[1993. *L'esprit d'aujourd'hui*, Vol. 317.]

CHAPTER 17

A CONSIDERATION ON THE WOLF MAN'S DREAM: FROM A KLEINIAN PERSPECTIVE

1. Introduction

It is considerably difficult to observe on the papers written by Freud, who is the founder of psychoanalysis and the most prominent researcher in its history, because many have already described their considerations and it is not easy to propose new perspectives. This is no exception for the paper on the case of Wolf Man. In that sense, it took a lot of courage to write this paper. In the field of ego psychology, the Wolf Man paper is highly evaluated for containing the most diverse elements of Freud's theories and perspectives including the importance of primal scene, research on infantile neurosis, the issue of castration complex and techniques for interpretation of the dream. The paper on Wolf Man is also introduced in the training for candidates as the most representative work of Freud's thoughts, which are written from a legitimate analytic perspective. I will, however, venture my personal opinion on such a classic paper, which will still be no more than a tentative assumption.

Applying the technique of dream interpretation, this paper analyses the meaning of the Wolf Man's dream from a view point of early object relation theory. It will especially consider the relationship between Wolf Man's therapeutic experiences or transferences and his dream at the time of therapy, which Freud did not mention. Wolf Man was 26 years old when he reported his dream.

2. Characteristics of the Wolf Man paper

It is safe to say that the Wolf Man paper develops the most complicated viewpoints among all Freud's clinical case reports. It has the following characteristics: 1) The case patient was consulted by Emil Kraepelin and diagnosed to have manic-depressive illness; however, modern diagnosis suggests that Wolf Man had a severe schizoid personality possessing a psychotic world characterized by apathy and withdrawal. 2) The limit setting psychotherapy was adopted. 3) The 25-year-old patient analysed his own dream he had when he was 4 years old, and Freud focused his research on infantile neurosis. Freud did not give any consideration on the meaning of the adult patient's dream. There seems to have been various actual reasons for this but Freud did not mention why. 4) Freud highlighted the importance of the primal scene and father complex, that is castration complex, in infancy. He explained dream interpretation mainly from this perspective, too. 5) Freud referred to the establishment process of infantile obsessive neurosis. 6) He explained the importance of childhood experience. 7) He referred to the formation of the perversion inclination. 8) The patient suffered a relapse and went into a psychotic state after completion of Freud's therapy and thus, underwent treatment again. 9) The patient lived long compared to Freud's other patients and spoke a lot about the experiences he had with Freud.

3. Theory and techniques of Kleinian dream interpretation

Naturally, Kleinian analysts put an emphasis on dream interpretation in clinical practice. While the technique is based on Freud's element analysis, their fundamental perspective of comprehension is based on early object relation theory. The goal for Kleinians is to understand the object relations, defence mechanisms and various anxieties related to the paranoid-schizoid position and depressive position. In particular, Kleinians conduct interpretation focusing on the transference relation with the therapist.

4. Wolf Man's dream

The patient was 26 years old when he received dream analysis, although he had started receiving therapy from Freud at the age of 23 after a few years of withdrawal. The patient hardly spoke even after therapy started and analytic self-understanding did not deepen for three and a half years, so Freud suggested a limit setting of one year. From that day forward, the patient developed many associations and dream interpretations. The dream he had was a reminiscence of a dream he had when he was 4 years old. It was a dream of Christmas Eve, which was also his birthday. He went to bed in dismay for he thought the presents he got were not enough to celebrate his double anniversary and had the dream on that night. The dream was as follows:

> "I dreamt that it was night and that I was lying in bed. (My bed stood with its foot towards the window; in front of the window there was a row of old walnut trees. I know it was winter when I had the dream, and night-time.) Suddenly the window opened of its own accord, and I was terrified to see that some white wolves were sitting on the big walnut tree in front of the window. There were six or seven of them. The wolves were quite white, and looked more like foxes or sheep-dogs, for they had big tails like foxes and they had their ears pricked like dogs when they pay attention to something. In great terror, evidently of being eaten up by the wolves, I screamed and woke up. My nurse hurried to my bed, to see what had happened to me. It took quite a long while before I was convinced that it had only been a dream; I had had such a clear and life-like picture of the window opening and the wolves sitting on the tree. At last, I grew quieter, felt as though I had escaped from some danger, and went to sleep again."

Focusing on the description that the wolves were motionless and only looked, Freud interpreted the issues including primal scene and fear of father.

5. Interpretation of the two fairy tales

Freud said that he examined this dream centring on the two fairy tales the patient mentioned and discussed the issues as fear of father, castration anxiety and primal scene. This paper will first similarly look at the meaning of these two fairy tales. In doing so, the meaning of the above dream will become apparent. Particularly, I would like to illustrate the dynamics of the transference relations at the time of therapy. As is stated above, this is the point that Freud did not deal with. Incidentally, the paper will proceed on the assumption that the two fairy tales are well known.

(1) Little Red Riding Hood

Mother tells Little Red Riding Hood to visit her ill Grandmother (a mother who needs care: Wolf Man's mother was inclined to ill health and always needed care). (There is a possibility that, from his childhood, Wolf Man regarded taking care of his sickly mother was obligatory.) Mother also warned Little Red Riding Hood not to loiter around and to specially watch out for the Wolf but Little Red Riding Hood forgets this and breaks her promise. The Wolf (the persecutory bad object: a mother) arrives at Grandmother's house beforehand, swallows her up and pretends to be her. This indicates that the terrifying aggressive mother appears and takes the place of the care-needing sickly Grandmother (the other aspect of a mother) because Little Red Riding Hood did not listen to Mother and broke her promise when she went to visit Grandmother. The Wolf had big eyes and big pointed ears (just like the wolves in Wolf Man's dream). The Wolf then attacks Little Red Riding Hood and eats her up. The theme of the first half of this fairy tale is the issue of such an oral aggressive mother and combined parents. The aggressive castrating aspect expresses a phallic destruction. At the same time, the image of the Wolf swallowing Grandmother into its stomach with its big mouth expresses the persecutory aspect of the mother. In other words, the Wolf can be regarded as the combined aggressive aspects of the parents.

Then a Hunter (the good father) comes by and cuts the Wolf (the bad mother)'s stomach open to rescue Little Red Riding Hood and Grandmother out. The Hunter puts rocks (an aggressive phallus) into the Wolf's stomach in place of them. The Wolf (the bad mother) wakes up and goes to a well to drink water but falls into it. The good father who gets rid of the bad fellow (the bad parents) plays an important role of rescuing the good child or the good object from the bad mother. It must be this theme of the latter half that wins children's hearts.

(2) The Wolf and the Seven Little Kids

This fairy tale concerns the absent mother. Mother goat goes shopping leaving the kids at home, so it is Mother who is in fault. Then, the Wolf appears. In other words, when Mother (the good object) becomes absent, Wolf who stands for the inner bad object (the inner bad mother) comes into the scene (The inner bad mother and father are projected.) Wolf (the bad object) is cunning and deceives the kids who were obeying their mother, and eats everybody but the youngest who escaped because it was hiding high in the wall clock. Mother comes home and the youngest kid is able to meet up with the Good Mother, so it could provide some comfort to the devastated Mother. The seven kids as a whole are in a sense, the self of a child. Not all were eaten by the sly object (projection of the inner bad mother) and a part was able to meet with the Good Mother who came back again. The youngest tells Mother the whole story and thinks with her how to rescue its siblings. This means that the youngest kid (the child) was not totally destroyed by the bad object and was able to meet with Good Mother, share her sorrows and worked together with her to get rid of the Wolf (the bad image of parents).

The clock the youngest kid was hiding in is a symbol of time and stands for the self who was able to wait patiently for Mother to come back. The clock was high on the wall to protect the kid from Wolf. In addition, inside the clock was such a place Wolf would never come up with to hide in, so the youngest was capable of deluding Wolf. It is interesting that, on his first clinical contact with Freud, Wolf Man was nervous about the wall clock in the consultation room. Wolf Man might have had a persecutory experience against Freud and phantasized himself hiding in the clock. Simply put, the kid (a part of the self of a child) who had firm secondary functions, such as time and space senses and thinking, was able to survive persecutory aggression. This implies that the part of self with adequate secondary functions can manage to survive such persecutory experiences. The survived part of self was able to meet up with the returned Good Mother, be a relief for her and even rescue its siblings (the other parts of self) with her. The imagination where the kids were rescued from the stomach of Wolf, who is a symbol of the terrifying combined parents, is a world of healthy omnipotent relief. The bad Wolf was finally disposed of by the returned Good Mother with the help of the kids' wisdom. This fairy tale is a syntonic world for children because everything happens in a magical world while the Wolf is asleep without him noticing.

6. Dream interpretation regarding transferences

Wolf Man's dream can be interpreted even only by analysing these two fairy tales and the context of the dream itself. There are few data left on the clinical course of Wolf Man so further dream interpretation will be implemented on an arbitrary analogy. Basically, the dream expresses a child's persecutory experience against an absent mother. When the mother goes away (or the child goes away from the mother), even on a temporary basis, and the child does not obey his/her mother or tries but fails, the bad mother object or probably the bad combined parents appear and eat the child. This is a representative of oral persecutory aggression and well displays the activity of the inner object. Then, the good father or good mother appears. The Hunter, who stands for the good father and the returned good mother, rescues the children trapped in the destructive world of the bad mother or combined parents (the Wolf's stomach) with their wisdom and power without the Wolf noticing. The bad object is therefore killed by the rocks (a destructive phallus of justice that punishes the bad) put in his stomach.

In this way, from the considerations of these two fairy tales alone, the themes of Wolf Man's dream can be analogized: mother absence, appearance of persecutory object (the bad mother or the bad combined parents), attack of being eaten, rescue due to the appearance of the good father or the good mother, and the punishment and destruction of the bad object. As is stated later, these have a deep correlation with the transference situation.

Freud also paid attention to the similarities of these two fairy tales. The similarities are that the main characters are eaten by the Wolf and are rescued out from the Wolf's stomach; the Wolf is put rocks in his stomach instead of them and dies in the end. For some reason, Freud focused especially on the description that the wolves in the Wolf Man's dream were staring and motionless. Freud took the meaning of the dream as fear of father and developed his theory in association with castration complex and primal scene.

Wolf Man's understanding of his childhood dream did not proceed for a long time until Freud proposed him a limit setting. Since then, Wolf Man positively spent his time to understand its meaning within the few months Freud had set. This is closely related to transference. There is little information about the then relation of Wolf Man and Freud, but therapy did not advance for several years because Wolf Man kept silence. It seems that it was a period when Freud underwent hard times and suffered from counter-transferences. Freud considered that he could not overlook Wolf Man's sabotage and declared to him that he would call off therapy, which had continued for three and a half years, after a year. From that day forward, the patient began to bring up abundant associations that promoted self-interpretation including the interpretation of the dream.

Considering the background, it can be well understood why Wolf Man began to work on his dream. Wolf Man felt that the therapist suddenly began to impose a strict rule and duty on him. He feared that if he could not obey the therapist, he would be swallowed and killed by the persecutory therapist just like the terrifying Wolf did in the two fairy tales. To run away from this situation, Wolf Man had no choice but to climb up a tree as the tailor did (this will be described later in this paper) or hide in a wall clock as the youngest kid did, but when the Wolf climbed after him, he had nowhere to escape. It is not surprising if the therapist waiting patiently to listen to him changed into an image of a therapist with fierce big eyes and mouth who intrudes into his world and destroys it with every tactic.

From a clinical course perspective, the description "Suddenly the window opened" expressed the experience where Wolf Man had no choice but to open the window of his mind or was forced to open it, and that his world was beginning to be intruded.

The dream also indicated a strong anticipation towards the therapist, that is, a good powerful man would appear and save him in the end. In this way, the Wolf Man's image of the therapist was split into two: a persecutory bad object and a good therapist who saves the patient in the end.

In his dream, Wolf Man thought the wolves were like foxes or dogs and was not completely afraid of them. This implied that Wolf Man's image of the therapist, Freud, was not a totally bad one and that he saw a good object world in the background.

Freud concentrated in considering infantile neurosis when Wolf Man had this dream, however, this paper will rather focus on the here and now experiences such as the transference relation the adult Wolf Man experienced at the therapeutic site.

7. Element association of Wolf Man's other dreams

(1) When Wolf Man was little, his big sister often used to show him the illustration of the wolf in the Little Riding Hood book and scare him, so Wolf Man had a wolf phobia. His big sister committed suicide when he was 19 years old.
(2) About the colour "white". When Wolf Man was living in a suburban residence in his childhood, his father kept white sheep. Father was proud of the sheep and often showed them to Wolf Man, but one day most of them died because of an epidemic and even more died when specialists tried to cure them. It is possible that this happened on the day before of Wolf Man's fourth birthday.
(3) Wolf Man told the following story: A tailor cut the tails of the wolves that came in from a window. The tailor met again with the pack of wolves in the forest so he climbed up a tree to escape. The wolves rode piggybacks on each other to reach the tailor but the tailor threatened them that he would cut their tails again. The wolves got scared and lost their balance so the tailor succeeded in driving them away.

This paper will study these additional element associations as well as the interpretations of the two fairy tales. First, there is an association on his big sister who committed suicide around then. This big sister often used to scare Wolf Man by showing him pictures of wolves. The anger and destruction against her materialized by her suicide. This was a big incident concerning an ambivalent object loss.

Secondly, he experienced object loss for his father who also died around then suffering from manic depressive illness. Wolf Man must have felt that his father's illness deteriorated not only because his father felt totally disappointed to lose his sheep one after another just before the 4-year-old Wolf Man had the dream, but also because the support from specialists made the results worse. His father eventually committed suicide when Wolf Man was 21 years old. It seems that Wolf Man possessed strong distrust, dissatisfaction and anger against the doctors who could not save his father.

Wolf Man became depressed when he was 18, and his sister and father died when he was 19 and 21 years old, respectively. Wolf Man's symptoms never improved until he consulted Freud at the age of 23.

This also suggests Wolf Man's transference to Freud. It is possible that Freud, who strongly tried to instigate treatment by fixing a limit setting for the end of therapy, stimulated the pathology world of Wolf Man's object loss. Since specialists killed his father's precious sheep, his father's manic-depressive illness worsened, prolonged and in the end he died without recovery. Wolf Man feared he would suffer the same problems as his father, that is, his medical conditions would worsen and he would have to leave Freud without being saved and die just like his sister and father.

The story of the tailor expressed the images of the father and therapist who disposed of the bad wolf (the bad mother). The wolves who were cut their tails expressed a castrated woman. The previous bad aggressive mother is a mother incorporated with a destructive phallus of the father. When the tailor (therapist) was attacked again by the bad wolves (the bad mother), he succeeded in escaping from them by threatening them that they did not possess aggressive powerful phalluses anymore. The tailor indicated the therapist who could successfully ward off the attack of such an aggressive bad mother or combined parents and protect Wolf Man.

8. The fairy tales and family image

The characters such as Mother, Grandmother, Mother goat and Wolf who appear in the two fairy tales in Wolf Man's dream seem to reflect his image of parents effectively. The image can be known by analogy through the description of his family situation when the 4-year-old Wolf Man had this dream. Freud just understood the family image with the father in the centre by focusing on fear of father, castration complex and especially on primal scene. He also mentioned about Wolf Man's mother sometimes and devoted many pages to the women who lived with the patient such as his sister, who is thought to have been a deputy of his mother, his nanny and his tutor. However, Freud emphasized that these women just provided traumatic experiences of sexual temptation. From another viewpoint, these women are described also as persecutory objects; expect for his nanny who protected him kindly, according to the description. Freud could not place the issue of mother or women at his theoretical centre.

Wolf Man's parents were prone to illness and often went on a trip leaving Wolf Man and his sister at home with their nanny and tutor. His mother, who was a hypochondriac self-centred woman, was ill in bed most of the time because of a female genital disease; therefore, it seems that she could hardly look after him as a mother from his childhood. On the other hand, his father repeated prolonged stays in a sanatorium because of manic-depressive illness. Such experiences of detachment and deprivation from his sickly parents and agonizing experiences of object loss and separation triggered by his parents' and sister's illness and death casted a dark shadow on the family. They strongly effected Wolf Man and brought down pathologic influences on him. As is described above, Wolf Man's family history and family image had something in common with the themes of the two fairy tales: the sickly grandmother of Little Red Riding Hood, the absent father of the seven little kids and the wolf that symbolizes an oral destructive mother.

The miserable mother who lost her daughter and husband remained neurotic even after Wolf Man became an adult and only talked about money to him. The trigger for the patient's illness was gonorrhoea. This indicated a pathological identification with the symptoms of the genital disease of his mother, whom was in an ambivalent relation with Wolf Man. Of course, there were the issues of onset and the subsequent death of his father and sister in the background. Freud also discussed the identification with his mother and his desire to be incorporated into her body or return to her uterus. However, Freud considered the pathological identification occurred only for Wolf Man to acquire a world of sexual experience with his father, and treated the matter as negative Oedipus complex.

Nevertheless, Wolf Man probably mundanely experienced that his sickly, selfish, and often absent mother, just as the mothers in the fairy tales, turned into a persecutory aggressive bad mother in his inner phantasy world. This can also be said about his father who was repeatedly hospitalized and often absent, therefore the combined parents seem to have had a big impact on Wolf Man as a persecutory bad object.

9. Conclusion

Freud emphasized the importance of infantile neurosis, castration complex and primal scene on the Wolf Man case.

This paper considered the issue of transference towards the therapist, which Freud did not mention much about. It illustrated the here and now transference relation with the therapist by taking a look at the meaning of Wolf Man's dream associations, which are the fairy tales of Little Red Riding Hood and The Wolf and the Seven Little Kids, the fact that his big sister used to frighten him with the wolves in a picture book, the mass death of his father's precious sheep, and the story of the tailor and the wolf. Furthermore, I described that the image of Wolf Man's family and his family history have a certain correspondence with the object relations indicated in the two fairy tales.

References

(1) Azuma, Yukari and Myoki, Hiroyuki, ed. 1993. "Freud's Cases". *L'esprit d'aujourd'hui*, Vol. 317 (in Japanese)

(2) Freud, Sigmund. 1918. "From the History of an Infantile Neurosis". In *Standard Edition*, Vol. 17. London: Hogarth Press.

(3) Kanzer, Mark and Glenn, Jules. 1980. *Freud and His Patients*. Lanham: Janson Aronson.

(4) Kinugasa, Takayuki. 1991. "Dream Theory in Object Relation". *Imago*, Extra Edition "Dreams", Vol. 2-12 (in Japanese)

(5) Kinugasa, Takayuki. 1997. "Analysis of Dreams: Development from Klein to Bion". *L'esprit d'aujourd'hui*, Extra Issue "Analysis of dreams" (in Japanese)

(6) Kinugasa, Takayuki. 1998. "Everyday Analysis and Dream Interpretation". *The Japanese journal of psycho-analysis*, Vol. 42, No. 3: 276-283 (in Japanese) (Chapter 15 in this book (in English))